The Concise Book of Dry Needling

The Concise Book of Dry Needling

Practical Applications for Myofascial Trigger Point Therapy

JOHN SHARKEY

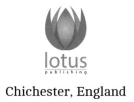

lotus
publishing

Chichester, England

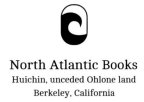

North Atlantic Books
Huichin, unceded Ohlone land
Berkeley, California

First published in 2016, and redesigned in 2024 by
Lotus Publishing
Apple Tree Cottage, Inlands Road, Nutbourne, Chichester, PO18 8RJ, and
North Atlantic Books
Huichin, unceded Ohlone land
Berkeley, California

All Drawings Amanda Williams
Photographs Laura Connick and Karen Cosgrave
Text Design Medlar Publishing Solutions Pvt Ltd., India
Cover Design Chris Fulcher
Printed and Bound Kultur Sanat Printing House, Turkey

The Concise Book of Dry Needling: Practical Applications for Myofascial Trigger Point Therapy is sponsored and published by North Atlantic Books, an educational non-profit based on the unceded Ohlone land Huichin (Berkeley, CA), that collaborates with partners to develop cross-cultural perspectives, nurture holistic views of art, science, the humanities, and healing, and seed personal and global transformation by publishing work on the relationship of body, spirit, and nature.

North Atlantic Books' publications are distributed to the US trade and internationally by Penguin Random House Publishers Services. For further information, visit our website at www.northatlanticbooks.com.

Medical Disclaimer: This book is intended for the purpose of providing an easy-to-reference resource to suitably qualified therapists for whom dry needling is within their scope of practice. Professional training leading to a recognized qualification in myofascial trigger point dry needling is essential.

Acknowledgment: I wish to acknowledge the support and input of Cristopher Alejandro (M.Sc. neuromuscular therapist/chartered physiotherapist). Special thanks to models Karen Cosgrave and Laura Connick.

British Library Cataloguing-in-Publication Data
A CIP record for this book is available from the British Library
ISBN 978 1 905367 67 2 (Lotus Publishing)
ISBN 978 1 62317 083 7 (North Atlantic Books)

Library of Congress Cataloguing-in-Publication Data
Names: Sharkey, John, 1961- author. | Society for the Study of Native Arts
    and Sciences, sponsoring body.
Title: The concise book of dry needling : practical applications for
    myofascial trigger point therapy / John Sharkey.
Description: Berkley, California : North Atlantic Books, 2016. | Includes
    bibliographical references and index.
Identifiers: LCCN 2016015020 (print) | LCCN 2016015990 (ebook) |
    ISBN 9781623170837 (pbk.) | ISBN 9781623170844 (ebook)
Subjects: | MESH: Myofascial Pain Syndromes--therapy | Acupuncture Therapy |
    Trigger Points
Classification: LCC RM184 (print) | LCC RM184 (ebook) | NLM WE 550 |
    DDC 615.8/92--dc23
LC record available at https://lccn.loc.gov/2016015020

Foreword

I wish to include a few words from the father of myofascial trigger points, the late David G. Simons. He wrote these words in 2008 for my first book on the topic, *The Concise Book of Neuromuscular Therapy*; his comments are noteworthy, because they are as applicable today as they were when he first wrote them.

'Although my career has been focused on myofascial trigger points and encouraging health care professionals to integrate them into their clinical thinking and practice, I am constantly reminded of the importance of fitting this specialized knowledge into the big picture. Understanding muscle structure and function is essential for the most effective identification and treatment of muscle pain and dysfunctions.'

'John has emphasized this important information in this volume. However, what we need to investigate next stems from the fact that the trigger point manuals are only half of the myofascial trigger point story. This is of fundamental importance. The manuals are focused on the pain caused by active myofascial trigger points: the effect of active myofascial trigger points on the sensory nervous system.

What is now becoming apparent is that myofascial trigger points can produce equally potent effects and disturbances in the motor nervous system, causing weakness due to muscle inhibition in the same or other muscles, loss of coordination, and sometimes reflex spasm in other muscles. These distant effects are just about as consistent for a particular myofascial trigger point location and have as much individually variability as referred pain patterns but are a much different and largely unexplored story.'

'Clinical myofascial pain, by definition, comes from active myofascial trigger points. Noteworthy, motor disturbances, which usually have no corresponding pain symptoms, are more likely to arise from pain-asymptomatic latent myofascial trigger points that until recently were generally considered just therapeutic red herrings.'

'You have my heartfelt best wishes for a successful career in this remarkably challenging field.'

David G. Simons, M.D. (1922–2010)

Dedication

This book is dedicated to David G. Simons

With love to Fidelma, Xsara, and Katie

Contents

Foreword   5
Preface   11

Introduction   **13**
Pain—Present, Past, Future   13
"X" Does Not Mark the Spot   14
Biotensegrity and Dry Needling   15
The Cellular Level   16
Understanding Anatomy   18
Why Consider Myofascial Trigger Point Dry
    Needling in the Treatment of Chronic
    Myofascial Pain?   19
Can Acupuncturists Perform Myofascial
    Trigger Point Dry Needling?   20

PART I   THEORY AND PRACTICE

Chapter 1
**Genesis of the Myofascial
Trigger Point**   **24**
Contractions—Pulling It All Together   27
A New Hypothesis   30

Chapter 2
**Standards and Guidelines in Myofascial
Trigger Point Dry Needling**   **31**
Anatomical Excellence   31
General Standards and Guidelines—
    Pre-treatment   31
General Standards and Guidelines—
    Post-treatment   32
General Standards and Guidelines—
    During Treatment   32
Risks and Cautions in Myofascial
    Trigger Point Dry Needling   33
Contraindications to Myofascial
    Trigger Point Dry Needling   34
Ruling Out Visceral Pain—
    "When in Doubt, Refer"   34
Before Starting—The Ten-Point Guidelines   36
A Few Words About Dietary Influences   36
Needle Application   37
Health and Safety Considerations   38

Chapter 3
**Central Sensitization and Control
of Perpetuating Factors**   **41**
Spinal Facilitation   42
Keys to Symptom Management   44

Initiating, Aggravating, and
  Perpetuating Factors   44
Perpetuating Factor Types: A Long
  Short War   45
Examples   45

Chapter 4
**Treatment Options and Chronic
Pain Management**   **51**
Stretch and Spray—Active Cold Therapy
  Stretching   51
A Note on Palpation   52
Chronic Pain Management—
  Three Key Steps   52
Medications   56

PART II   MAJOR SKELETAL MUSCLES AND REFERRED PAIN PATTERNS

Chapter 5
Muscles of the Face, Head, and Neck   **58**
Occipitofrontalis   58
Temporalis   60
Masseter   62
Pterygoids   64
Platysma   66
Hyoids   67
Digastricus   70
Longus colli   71
Longus capitis   73
Rectus capitis (anterior, lateralis)   74
Scalenes   76
Sternocleidomastoid   78
Rectus capitis posterior (major, minor)   81
Obliquus capitis inferior   82
Obliquus capitis superior   83

Chapter 6
Muscles of the Trunk and Spine   **84**
Erector spinae (sacrospinalis)   84
Splenius capitis   87
Splenius cervicis   88
Longissimus capitis   90
Multifidus   92
Rotatores   94
Intercostals   95
Diaphragm   97
Internal oblique   98
External oblique   99
Transversus abdominis   101
Rectus abdominis   102
Psoas major   104
Iliacus   106
Psoas minor   107
Quadratus lumborum   108

Chapter 7
**Muscles of the Shoulder
and Upper Arm**   **110**
Trapezius   110
Rhomboids   113
Pectoralis minor   114
Supraspinatus   116
Infraspinatus   117
Teres minor   119
Subscapularis   121
Teres major   123
Serratus anterior   124
Levator scapulae   126
Pectoralis major   127
Subclavius   129
Latissimus dorsi   130
Deltoid   133
Biceps brachii   135
Coracobrachialis   136
Brachialis   138
Triceps brachii   139
Anconeus   141

Chapter 8

Muscles of the Forearm and Hand   143

Pronator teres   143
Forearm flexors   144
Adductor pollicis   147
Abductor pollicis longus   148
Pronator quadratus   149
Abductor pollicis brevis   150
Abductor digiti minimi   151
Brachioradialis   152
Extensor carpi radialis brevis   153
Extensor carpi radialis longus   154
Extensor digitorum   155
Flexor carpi ulnaris   157
Supinator   158
Opponens pollicis   160
Palmaris longus   161

Chapter 9

Muscles of the Hip and Thigh   163

Gluteus maximus   163
Gluteus medius   165
Gluteus minimus   167
Tensor fasciae latae   168
Piriformis   169
Gemelli   171
Obturator internus   172
Obturator externus   173

Quadratus femoris   174
Adductor longus   176
Adductor magnus   177
Adductor brevis   179
Gracilis   180
Pectineus   181
Hamstrings   182
Sartorius   185
Quadriceps   186

Chapter 10

Muscles of the Leg and Foot   189

Gastrocnemius   189
Tibialis anterior   191
Flexor digitorum longus   193
Flexor hallucis longus   194
Extensor hallucis longus   195
Tibialis posterior   196
Popliteus   197
Fibularis longus   199
Plantaris   201
Soleus   202
Abductor hallucis   204
Adductor hallucis   205

Glossary   *207*
Bibliography   *213*

Preface

This text concerns the treatment of myofascial trigger points through the exclusive use of *dry needling*, a term coined by Dr. Janet Travell in the famous "big red books" (Simons, Travell, and Simons 1999, pp. 154–155). Dry needling (with the use of a fine filament needle) is the ideal tool for therapists, of every stripe, involved in treating myofascial trigger points in adults, provided it falls within their scope of practice.

The book is written in a concise manner as a "quick-to-hand" reference guide regarding key issues around safe, effective, and appropriate dry needling. It is intended to be the ideal accompaniment to course notes and the perfect in-office tableside reference guide. Accurate and essential criteria are provided for the identification and subsequent treatment of myofascial trigger points through the exclusive use of a fine, filiform needle. Skilled palpation, supported by the ability to visualize and observe anatomical landmarks, is essential to avoid neurovascular and other vital structures that could result in insult, injury, or additional pain.

A description of the origin, etiology, and pathophysiology of the myofascial trigger point is offered. Indications and contraindications for myofascial trigger point dry needling are noted, and standards and guidelines are presented. Images concerning correct needle application/insertion are supplied for many muscles in the body, while guidelines are provided for muscles that are in the proximity of the ones chosen for inclusion in the photographs. Two bespoke myofascial trigger point hypotheses concerning the mechanism of myofascial trigger points, along with the rationale for the success of dry needling, are also presented for further consideration and research.

This text does not deal with acupuncture or the many refined techniques and diverse approaches of that discipline; it focuses solely on the use of dry needling for the exclusive treatment of myofascial trigger points. The book is not a substitute for understanding the neurophysiological mechanisms of local or referred pain, or for completing an appropriate course of study in dry needling. Such a course should be delivered by a recognized, competent training provider who understands their responsibility to learners, which includes legal, ethical, and professional knowledge.

This book is intended for use by suitably and adequately qualified therapists as a quick-reference tool. This book is not about personal opinions but is about best practice.

Illustrations and More

Images of dry needling application have been provided throughout for the reader's convenience. Images are not necessary for all muscles, especially for muscles in the forearm, as the needling procedures are so similar. The guidelines for needle application may be much the same for a muscle within the proximity of the ones chosen for image capture. Care is therefore required when changing the angle or needle direction, keeping in mind the need to ensure appropriate depth while recognizing anatomical location. For the purposes of clarity, in a selected number of the photographs, a delivery tube or black line replaces the needle to more clearly show the needle application.

Do not attempt to offer dry needling unless you have received appropriate training from a recognized training provider. You do not need to have received training, however, to enjoy the book or to learn about myofascial trigger points.

However, I wish to pay tribute to authors Jan Dommerholt and César Fernández-de-las-Peñas for producing the only other book (at the time of writing) on this specific topic—Trigger Point Dry Needling—published in 2013. Their text is one that I recommend to everyone interested in the wider "potentially contentious issues" (as remarked by Leon Chaitow in the book's foreword). The book provides a platform for bridging the various disciplines involved in the wide range of needling techniques.

Please share this book with other therapists, medical practitioners, movement therapists, and others.

For more recent research and case study reports, see Kietrys, Palombaro, and Mannheimer (2014); Skorupska et al. (2014); and Cotchett, Munteanu, and Landorf (2014).

Introduction

Pain—Present, Past, Future

Pain is a liar; however, research has changed the way we think about pain (Moseley 2012). Pain is a child of the brain—to fully understand it we must meet the entire pain family. Peripheral tissues are close relations and could be viewed as brothers and sisters, while tissues such as muscle fibers and sarcomeres would be first cousins. Mechanoreceptors, proprioceptors, and nociceptors might be the irritated family members, constantly taking information to and from mom and dad concerning irritating older siblings. These various members of the family can have a tendency to exaggerate or distort the truth. For example, mom and dad can overreact, underreact, or misread the situation, dishing out a response that is disproportionate and not appropriate to the reality; this is ultimately referred to as "allodynia."

Chronic pain states are defined by significant changes in neuronal activity; such changes are profoundly influential in pain matrix mechanisms. Neuroplastic changes occur in the spinal cord, thalamic nuclei, cortex, and limbic system, and can alter pain thresholds, degree of sensitivity to pain, and the overall pain experiences of our patients (Woolf 2010).

Research by Staud (2011) describes spinal segmental sensitization (SSS) as being caused by heightened dorsal horn activity, brought about by constant bombardment of nociceptor impulses from the periphery (due to damaged or sensitized somatic or visceral tissues). Clinical experience of thousands of practicing therapists across the globe identifies pain referral patterns that cannot be of nerve origin. Travell and Simons (1992) reported myofascial trigger points within the soleus muscle that refer deep pain to the ipsilateral sacroiliac joint. Additional myofascial trigger points in the soleus refer exceptional pain to the face and jaw. Some mechanism or mechanisms other than nerve pathways must be at play in such situations, as nerves exclusively refer pain inferiorly (the face is the exception).

Far too few therapists and medical doctors are aware of the perpetuating role of myofascial trigger points as a combining source of sensory bombardment (Shah and Gilliams 2008), with the possible result of chronic pain in various guises. Myofascial pain, according to Fogelman and Kent (2015), is an "eminently treatable condition" yet almost "universally underdiagnosed by physicians and undertreated by physical therapy modalities." Constant noxious bombardment of the dorsal horn neuron causes a release of glutamate and substance P at the segmental level. By binding to their respective receptors on post-synaptic neurons, these chemicals induce sensitization of wide dynamic range (WDR) neurons, thus further sensitizing adjacent spinal segments. The sustained release of glutamate and substance P leads to apoptosis (programmed cell death) of inhibitory neurons. This perturbation leads to a sustained sensitized state, which in turn lowers neuronal pain thresholds, activates previously inactive synapses (expansion of the receptive field of pain), and leads to allodynia and hyperalgesia (Shah and Gilliams 2008).

Central sensitization that is maintained by myofascial trigger points and other peripheral sources can be reversed over time. Myofascial trigger point dry needling has been shown to be effective in that regard and therefore a worthwhile therapeutic intervention (Srbely et al. 2010). A more recent study measuring the concentrations of a diversity of biochemicals—including β-endorphin, substance P, tumor necrosis factor-α, cyclo-oxygenase-2, hypoxia-inducible factor 1-alpha, inducible nitric oxide synthase, and vascular endothelial growth factor—found that dry needling of trigger points modulates the concentrations of these noxious chemicals in a dosage-dependent manner (Hsieh et al. 2011).

Pain can have a crepuscular aspect to it. Time can also be a healer. However, chronic myofascial pain patients know all too well the feeling of misery and despair when neither time nor medication reduces the untiring relentlessness of pain or changes in sensation.

With its clear images concerning the correct use of needles, needle placement, and needle direction, this book will help ensure safe, effective, and appropriate clinical applications of myofascial trigger point dry needling, eradicating pain in the present and into the future; pain will become a past and distant memory or be reduced to manageable levels.

A paper in 1979 by Karl Lewit investigating the needle effect in the relief of myofascial pain reported that "dry needling is highly effective in the therapy of chronic myofascial pain. Immediate analgesia without hyperesthesia (the needle effect) can be produced by needling precisely the most painful spot."

Note: When I refer to *pain*, this is taken to mean "pain and changes in sensations."

"X" Does Not Mark the Spot

The reader will notice that the artwork in this book has no "X" to mark the position of the myofascial trigger point. This is because it is not appropriate to place an X in a specific position to identify the location of the myofascial trigger point. The point of view that the X represents a common location specific to a particular muscle is, in my opinion, a flawed argument, as thousands of therapists worldwide working daily with myofascial trigger points will attest. The latest third edition of Travell, Simons, and Simons *Myofascial Pain and Dysfunction* does not include diagrams with an "X" anymore and has adopted the stance promoted by Sharkey (2008) which was the first text to abandon the use of an "X."

Using an anatomical image with an "X" to identify the location of the myofascial trigger point is a poor substitute for excellent palpation skills. Such skills are essential for identifying the myofascial trigger point(s) that could be located *anywhere* in the hundreds of thousands of myofibrils in any one muscle. Appropriate palpation skills and knowledge of the cardinal signs are used to seek out the accompanying tense bands and nodules associated with myofascial trigger points, which are housed in the microscopic sarcomeres.

Biotensegrity and Dry Needling

My work in anatomy, physiology, and bodywork therapy has been significantly influenced by my mentor Stephen Levin M.D., an orthopedic surgeon who coined the term "biotensegrity." Dr. Levin promoted the biotensegrity model as the new biomechanics for all biological structures. Influenced by the work of Harvard University researcher Dr. Donald Ingber I describe tensegrity as "anatomy for the 21st century."

Tensegrity has emerged as the most significant development in human anatomy in recent years, with important ramifications for a wide range of medical practitioners, including surgeons, bio-engineers, and human

movement specialists. Bespoke Thiel soft-fix dissection techniques are providing a new vision and understanding of the continuity of the human form. A fresh look at human fascia highlights its role in providing continuous tension throughout its network.

The term tensegrity was coined by Buckminster Fuller by combining the words "tension" and "integrity." Fuller's student Kenneth Snelson built the first floating compression structure of tensegrity in 1949, while Dr. Stephen Levin was the pioneer of "biotensegrity," which was born out of his publications on the topic in the early 1970s (figure 0.1). As a clinical anatomist, I have investigated this model and the role of fascia in my dissections to better understand the mechanisms of human movement and chronic pain, while providing new anatomical

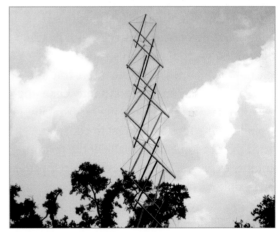

Figure 0.1. Using tensioned wire and metal struts, self-supporting structures can be created. The integrity of the structure requires the interplay between the compression and tension elements. As Snelson points out, however, while the breaking of one element in a simple structure can lead to its collapse, the challenging of one area in more complex constructions will be less catastrophic (for more, see his website, http://kennethsnelson.net/faq).

knowledge and awareness, leading to less invasive surgical and non-surgical therapeutic interventions.

Borrowing from Fuller's term "tensegrity," Levin added the prefix "bio," which refers to all living structures. Biotensegrity is the application of Fuller's tensegrity concepts to biological structure and physiology. In the biotensegrity model the limbs are not a collection of rigid body segments: the upper and lower limbs are semi-rigid, nonlinear, viscoelastic bony segments. These segments are interconnected by nonlinear, viscoelastic connectors, including cartilage, joint capsules, and ligaments, and have an integrated nonlinear, viscoelastic active motor system—the muscles, tendons, and fascia (connective tissue).

Biotensegrity counters the notion that the skeleton provides a frame for the soft tissues to hang upon; instead, biotensegrity structures are integrated, pre-tensioned (self-tensioned), continuous myofascial networks with floating discontinuous compression struts (the skeleton) contained within them. A column whose center of gravity is constantly changing while its base is rapidly moving horizontally would require forces too great to consider. The forces become incalculable if the column comprises several rigid bodies, hinged together by flexible, virtually frictionless, joints.

Daniele-Claude Martin, a pioneer in the world of biotensegrity and a member of the Biotensegrity Interest Group (B.I.G.), co-authored a chapter with Dr. Levin in the excellent book *Fascia: The Tensional Network of the Human Body* (Schleip et al. 2012). The title of the chapter was "Myofascia as the tensioner in the biotensegrity model," and Levin and Martin made the following important points regarding tension:

'Central to this concept is the understanding that the fascia imparts a continuous tension to the system. Fascia displays the nonlinearity characteristic of all biologic tissues. In nonlinear tissues, the stress/strain relationship never reaches zero (a characteristic of linear materials); and there is always tension inherent in the system. It gives the 'continuous tension,' an essential component of tensegrity, that helps set the tone of the organism. There are active contractile elements in fascia (Schleip et al. 2012) and the fascial network is intimately bound to muscle (Passerieux et al. 2007). Muscle also has intrinsic "tone" and is never completely lax, and the entire fascial network is continually tensed, by both intrinsic tension and active contractions that can be "tuned."'

This concept of tuning the fascia blends well with the fascial response to needles, as described by the neuroendocrinologist Helene Langevin. In her 2006 paper, entitled "*Connective tissue: A body-wide signaling network?*", Langevin detected a mechanical response whereby the connective tissue wrapped itself around the needle, with a resulting electrical signal being transmitted to the surrounding connective tissue cells via mechanotransduction. The change in tissue tension is obvious as the connective tissue swirls around the needle, creating a redistribution of tension and compression (biotensegrity).

The Cellular Level

At the cellular level, using fluoroscopic imaging Guimberteau et al. (2010) provided strong visual evidence that fascia contains a water-filled vacuolar system that is capable of sliding (I suggest "gliding") independently of the rate of contraction of muscle. In turn, it is capable of facilitating and supporting capillaries throughout the fascia.

Sharkey (2015) provided fresh-frozen cadaver images of the fascia profundus at the macro level which reflect this fractal microvacuolar structure while revealing an icosahedron-like (tensegrity) composition in which fractal elements inter-relate, creating a body-wide framework or network (figure 0.2).

This structure is able to change or maintain shape and form within a fluid base, allowing deformation and a subsequent return to its original state while maintaining volume. This creates the stable, yet flexible, environment necessary for fascia to act as a medium for force transmission (Huijing 2009).

This new model for biological structures that is based on the concept of Fasciategrity, a new portmanteau combining fascia research and tensegrity science first used by Sharkey and Avison, identifies fascia as the tensional, continuous member which includes bone as a specialized fascia on a spectrum of stiffness to softness (Sharkey, 2021). In a Fasciategrity model, continuous tensile forces (from the myofascial tissues) provide an "ocean" within which the struts float (in the human body, the "struts" are the bones, which are continuous, as bones are considered fascia, and do not directly transmit compression forces to each other). The tensional members are continuous and directly distribute their tensional load to all other tensional members, as described by Fuller in 1961 (figure 0.3).

The fascial oceans become seas, lakes, rivers, streams, and brooks; skin and bone represent opposite seashores. Newtonian, Hookian, and linear mechanical properties are the basis for the building of all things non-biological (Levin 1995). This description supports the more recently accepted image of a continuous tissue, ubiquitous in nature, connecting left to right, front to back, and top to bottom,

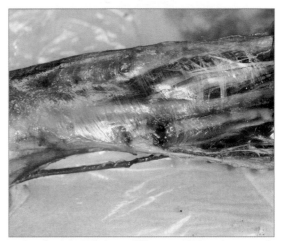

Figure 0.3. This amazing image illustrates the omnidirectional tensional network that is fascia. Even the muscle fibers are a specialized form of fascia. The absence of one precise vector allows maximum adaptation of the structure in a continuous evolution of balance through tensional and compressional forces. This is the fascial chaos of which my colleague Jean Claude Guimberteau speaks so eloquently. (Photograph: J. Sharkey 2010).

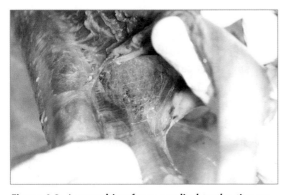

Figure 0.2. A stretching force applied to the tissues of the anterior forearm, on a fresh-frozen cadaveric specimen highlights the fractal, chaotic arrangement of the deep fascia. (Photograph: J. Sharkey 2010).

embracing and permeating the entire body (figure 0.4). Mesenchymal-derived connective tissues provide a body-wide network of communication (Schleip and Müller 2013).

Myofascial trigger point dry needling can furnish a mechanism to restore the fascial tone, so vital to the biotensegrity, providing

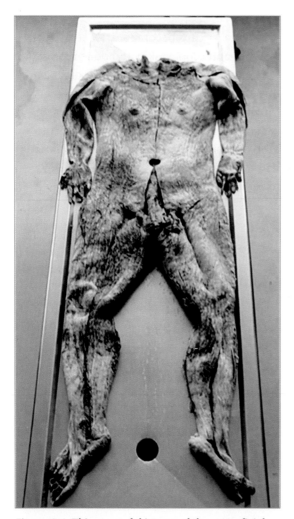

Figure 0.4. This powerful image of the superficial fascia, removed as one continuous structure, allows the dry needling myofascial trigger point therapist to imagine the fascial continuity and ubiquitous nature of this all-embracing tissue. (Photograph: J. Sharkey 2010).

a return to homeostasis, and thereby normalizing the tissues associated with, and connecting to, the myofascial trigger point. In fact, the muscle fiber within which is housed the myofascial trigger point is itself a specialization of fascia. Muscle fibers are part of a continuum of specialty that includes all the tissues of what Stephen Levin and Graham Scarr have called the "mesokinetic system."

Understanding Anatomy

I cannot overstate the need for an excellent understanding of anatomy, including surface, topographical, and gross anatomy. Taking time to become accustomed to the various lengths of the needles, coupled with the ability to visualize the needle once it has been placed in the tissue, will prove to be a vital skill. With an excellent knowledge of anatomy, I suggest it is virtually impossible to cause harm or injury to a patient. With a poor knowledge of anatomy, on the other hand, it will be only a matter of time before harm and injury comes to the patient. Know your anatomy.

As an exercise physiologist, I struggled with Travell and Simon's proposal that common myofascial trigger points can have their location identified by placing an "X" over specific locations of a given muscle. For example, in Volume 1 of the famous red books (Simons, Travell, and Simons 1999, p. 331), Barbara Cummings' images of the masseter muscle include several chunky "Xs" marking the positions of specific myofascial trigger points. The size of each "X" is such that if one superimposes all the images, the "Xs" cover the entire muscle. One "X" alone is covering tens of thousands of superficial to deep fibers.

In my daily work I speak to therapists who tell me that they could not find a myofascial trigger point in the middle of the most vertical fibers of the upper part of the trapezius muscle, as described on p. 279 of Simons, Travell, and Simons (1999). With appropriate palpation skills and the reassurance that the myofascial trigger point can form anywhere within the muscle, these same therapists further investigate and report they found the culprit distal, lateral, or superior to the location identified by the "X."

Using the Thiel soft-fix method of cadaveric dissection, I have demonstrated what I call "muscle islands." Muscle islands are small, isolated but regular, patches of muscle fibers or long thin cords of muscle fibers found on, or running in series with, muscle tendons (figure 0.5). These are, I believe, why therapists find and can irritate what are termed attachment trigger points. In fact, muscle islands can be found almost anywhere, especially in the subcutis, and represent what some researchers may call a panniculus effect. Dissection provides a very different reality of anatomy—one that is not as uniform or as ordered as one sees in the classical anatomy textbooks.

It should be noted that when dealing with a myofascial trigger point although the pleural is not often used you are in fact treating more than one myofascial trigger point, possibly dozens of myofascial trigger points or tens of dozens. Treating one muscle alone can be an exhaustive experience for the patient and hence why I recommend "less is more" especially when treating a new patient. I recommend minimizing the number of muscles treated to a maximum of three.

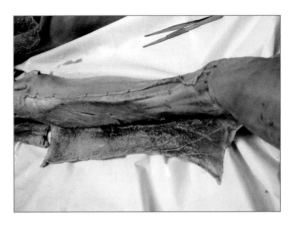

Figure 0.5. Image of a lower limb (anterior view) with the skin reflected, showing isolated muscles fibers just beneath the skin, or "muscle islands." (Photograph: J. Sharkey 2015).

Why Consider Myofascial Trigger Point Dry Needling in the Treatment of Chronic Myofascial Pain?

Myofascial pain arises from muscle and its connective tissue (Shah and Heimur 2012). According to Simons, Travell, and Simons (1999), and supported by numerous researchers over the preceding years (Mense 2010), myofascial trigger points are responsible for, or play a role in, as much as 85% of musculoskeletal pain. Myofascial trigger points constitute commonly overlooked or ignored causes of common musculoskeletal pain conditions, chronic or acute. My colleague and researcher Jay Shah has demonstrated that active myofascial trigger points have a noxious biochemical milieu—including substance P, bradykinins, and other substances—which is at the root of the pain. Many drug-based therapies have in fact been demonstrated to be no better than a placebo.

Recent research has suggested that ligand TRPV1 receptors and piezo channels may play a role in the development and maintenance of myofascial trigger points. TRPV1 receptors are located in sensory neurons and are activated by various stimuli, including heat, acid, and certain chemicals. Studies have shown that TRPV1 receptor expression is increased in myofascial trigger points and that activation of these receptors can lead to muscle pain and hyperalgesia (Yuan et al. 2021).

Piezo channels, on the other hand, are a type of mechanically activated ion channel found in various tissues, including muscle cells. Recent research has suggested that piezo channels may play a role in the development and maintenance of myofascial trigger points by sensitizing muscle cells to mechanical stimuli. Understanding the role of ligand TRPV1 receptors and piezo channels in myofascial trigger points could lead to the development of new therapies targeting these receptors and channels. For example, medications that block TRPV1 receptor activation or piezo channel sensitization could potentially reduce pain and dysfunction associated with myofascial trigger points. Based on this new research I recommend that light touch be introduced, if appropriate, as a preparation before needling as piezo channels open in response to light touch improving vascular blood supply a useful physiological response when providing dry needling.

A double-blind controlled dry needling study by Mayoral et al. (2013) demonstrated that the treatment of myofascial trigger points was superior to a placebo. In clinical practice, pain management or the eradication of pain is the primary focus for many patients and health care practitioners. It is worth noting that changes in sensation such as a constant itch, numbness, tingling, burning, crawling, or feelings of water running on the skin are all components across the spectrum of pain. These are real sensations that patients feel on an on-going daily basis—for some, twenty-four hours a day, every day. Not necessarily a pain per se, a change in sensation is rather a variation on the theme of pain.

A pain experienced radiating down the anterior upper limb and terminating in the wrist and palm connotes a brachial nerve insult. When all avenues of traditional medical assessment have been exhausted without identifying any underlying pathophysiological cause, or etiology, then soft tissue myofascial trigger points must be considered. Myofascial trigger points can mimic or play significant contributing roles in migraines, cervicogenic headaches, frozen shoulder and associated pain issues, carpal or tarsal tunnel syndromes, frozen or lower back pain, sciatic pain, radiculopathies, knee and ankle pain, and a host of other conditions. Put simply, myofascial trigger points can mimic anything. For those patients who have "tried everything" with little or no therapeutic benefit, myofascial trigger point dry needling is worth considering.

Can Acupuncturists Perform Myofascial Trigger Point Dry Needling?

Although acupuncture practitioners already possess excellent needle-handling skills, they will additionally require knowledge of the pathophysiology, etiology, and pain referral patterns of myofascial trigger points. They will also need to develop the palpation skills required to feel for and find and locate myofascial trigger points to ensure accuracy during dry needling application. Myofascial trigger points are not acupuncture points, tender points, or ah shi points, and can form anywhere in the millions of muscle fibers throughout the body. Overlapping acupuncture points with myofascial trigger points and then removing all but the points that coincide would obviously lead the uninitiated to see a corresponding relationship.

Central Vs. Attachment Trigger Points

As a clinical anatomist, I have investigated the idea of attachment trigger points and have arrived at the following proposal/suggestion. During dissection it is obvious that small clusters of isolated muscle fibers are found lying on the body of a tendon or on the undersurface of the skin throughout the body (figure 0.6). These muscle islands can by their very nature develop myofascial trigger points, thus leading to the notion of "attachment" trigger points.

Recommendation

Treat myofascial trigger points within the gasters of the muscles and then re-examine the attachment trigger points to see if they have dissipated after the primary source has been treated. Attachment trigger points are most often the offspring of the primary parent trigger points.

Myocardial Myofascial Trigger Points

Much research in this field still needs to be done. For example, no research currently exists concerning the possible existence and consequence of myocardial myofascial trigger points. I therefore call for and encourage research on this topic. I suspect that many people, convinced they have had or are having a coronary episode, suffer unnecessary stress/strain, when in fact they may be experiencing

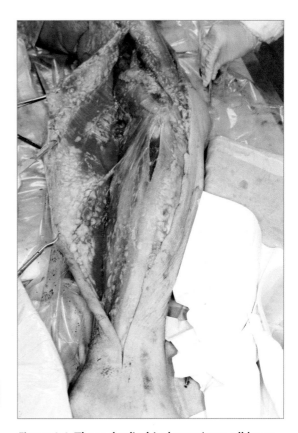

Figure 0.6. The red cylindrical protein we all know as muscle fibers can be found as muscle islands beneath the skin or on the outer surface of a tendon and can house myofascial trigger points. (Photograph: J. Sharkey 2010).

a myocardial myofascial trigger point. As the heart is a striated muscle, it seems logical that it conceivably harbors myofascial trigger points, and I would welcome research into this uncharted territory.

As I mentioned earlier, an appreciation concerning the role of ligand TRPV1 receptors and piezo channels in myofascial trigger points could lead to the development of new drug therapy targeting these receptors and channels and this would be a most welcomed development concerning treatment of myocardial myofascial trigger points.

PART I

THEORY AND PRACTICE

Genesis of the Myofascial Trigger Point

Myofascial trigger points are hyperirritable localized spots found in taut bands within the muscle sarcomeres (Simons, Travell, and Simons 1999). The hollow sarcoplasmic reticulum (SR) functions to store calcium ions that are constantly being pumped into it from the cytoplasm of the cell. When muscle fibers are not contracted, a high concentration of calcium is located in the sarcoplasmic reticulum, and low concentrations exist within the sarcoplasm. Special calcium gates can remain closed, blocking calcium from escaping and moving into the sarcoplasm. When an impulse travels along the membrane of the sarcoplasmic reticulum, these calcium gates open and allow a flood of calcium ions to rush out of the sarcoplasmic reticulum and into the sarcoplasm of the sarcomere, where the myofilaments are located. This is a key step in the normal sequence leading to muscle contractions.

Myofibrils consist of three types of myofilaments: "myosin," the thick protein; "actin," the thin protein; and "titan," the sticky protein. These myofilaments are arranged in a very precise pattern. The thick myofilaments are surrounded by six thin spiraling myofilaments, while the titan proteins act as tails to anchor the myosin to the Z disc. In figure 1.1, the thin actin myofilaments can be seen above and below each thick myofilament; in reality, however, they spiral around the thick proteins in a snakelike fashion.

It should be noted that research has confirmed several other proteins located within sarcomeres.

Some of these include:

1. Nebulin—a giant protein that runs parallel to actin filaments and regulates their length.
2. Tropomodulin—a protein that caps the pointed end of actin filaments and regulates their shape.
3. Tropomyosin—a protein that wraps around actin filaments and regulates the interaction between actin and myosin.
4. Myomesin—a protein that cross-links the M-lines of adjacent sarcomeres, providing stability to the sarcomere.

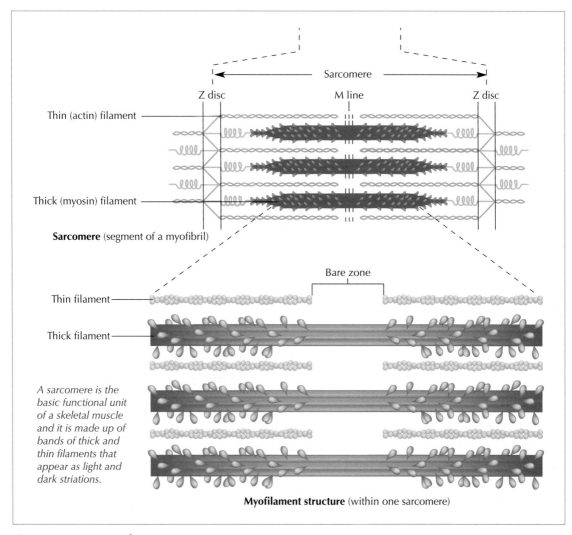

Figure 1.1. Structure of a sarcomere.

5. Obscurin—a giant protein that connects the Z-discs to the myosin thick filaments and plays a role in maintaining the structural integrity of the sarcomere.
6. C-protein—a protein that binds to the myosin thick filaments and helps regulate their shape and stability.
7. Alpha-actinin—a protein that cross-links actin filaments and anchors them to the Z-discs.

These proteins, along with actin, myosin, and titin, play important roles in the structure and function of sarcomeres, and their discovery has expanded our understanding of the molecular mechanisms that underlie muscle contraction and inhibition.

Within each sarcomere the myofilaments overlap, similarly to when the bristles of two brooms are pressed into each other

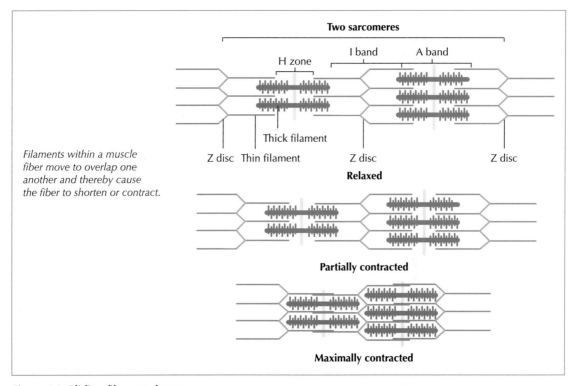

Filaments within a muscle fiber move to overlap one another and thereby cause the fiber to shorten or contract.

Figure 1.2. Sliding filament theory.

(figure 1.2). When viewed under a microscope, the ends of a sarcomere appear lighter than in the center; this is because the thick myofilaments are situated in the center, while the thin myofilaments are located toward the ends. The name "striated muscle" was used for this very reason. "I band" is the name given to the light areas, while the dark areas are called "A bands". Near the center of the "I band" is a thin dark line known as the "Z line" or "Z disc": the "Z line" is where sarcomeres come together, and the thin myofilaments of adjacent sarcomeres overlap slightly. The thick myofilament "myosin" has a core with heads that stick out like the head of a golf club (two heads actually); these are also referred to as "myosin cross bridges". These bridges or heads have some important characteristics:

- Adenosine triphosphate (ATP) binding sites
- Actin binding sites
- A hinge that allows a swiveling action so that the head can move the thin proteins, resulting in a contraction

Note the spherical shape of the long chains of actin molecules (also called "G actins"). The thin protein actin is constructed of two chains ("H" and "G" proteins) spiraling around each other. A smaller associated protein, "tropomyosin," in turn coils around the actin, as shown. Yet another protein, "troponin," attaches itself at specific intervals to the tropomyosin. As these proteins are electromagnetically attracted to each other, once the troponin moves it will in turn move the attached tropomyosin with it. Here is the important point: tropomyosin covers the binding sites on the actin, and when the tropomyosin is attracted away by the movement of those electrically charged proteins acting on the troponin, the sites become free for the cross heads (or bridges) of the electromagnetically charged thick myosin to attract and associate (glide). This is how a muscle contracts.

Contractions—Pulling It All Together

When muscles are working normally, they require a nerve impulse; this is the very first step leading to a contraction (figure 1.3).

This nerve impulse will travel along the sarcolemma and into the T tubules. From there the nerve impulse will travel to the sarcoplasmic reticulum, resulting in the active opening of the calcium gates, allowing calcium to diffuse into the sarcomeres, where the myofilaments are located. Calcium ions now bind to the troponin molecule, altering the shape of the protein and causing it to move, thereby moving the attached tropomyosin. Now that the tropomyosin has moved, the myosin binding sites become free, permitting the myosin heads to attach to and pull the actin. As the heads contact the actin, the myosin cross bridges hinge and swivel, thus pulling the myofilament actin; this does not

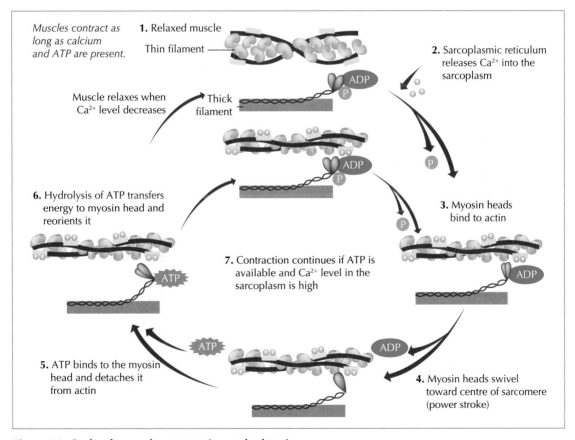

Figure 1.3. Cycle of muscular contraction and relaxation.

happen all at once, but in a way similar to a tug of war team pulling a rope.

The pulling action occurs in a synchronized manner: some myosin heads attach while others disassociate—a collective effort that leads to a concentric contraction. Should the external force overcome the pulling action, or should a person consciously allow the muscle to be overcome, the result is a lengthening of the muscle while it is pulling on the myofilaments; this is known as an "eccentric contraction." Remember, this means that muscles can only pull—they cannot push.

For muscles to work effectively, energy is required; this energy is supplied by the breakdown of ATP. As long as calcium remains in the presence of the myofilaments, the sarcomeres will remain shortened. Under normal circumstances, when the nerve impulse stops, the membrane of the sarcoplasmic reticulum is no longer permeable to calcium ions, and the calcium gates now act in reverse, allowing the calcium ions to escape from the sarcomere back into the sarcoplasmic reticulum. As the calcium disassociates from the troponin, it now pulls the tropomyosin back into its resting place covering the myosin binding sites. Tropomyosin then, once more, blocks the cross bridges from touching the thin actin protein, thus preventing a contraction from taking place.

From the above description of muscle contraction, the reader can appreciate that calcium is the "key" that turns on a contraction, or for that matter turns it off. If, for some reason, calcium ions cannot escape from the sarcomere (or, as proposed by Gerwin, Dommerholt, and Shah (2004), a damaged sarcoplasmic reticulum leads

to a flood of calcium concentrations), then the myofilaments will remain shortened. A dysfunctional endplate activity occurs, commonly associated with a strain (resulting from, for example, unaccustomed physical activity) or other soft tissue insult. Stored calcium ions are released at the site; acetylcholine (ACh) is released through calcium-charged gates at the synapse, leading to an abundant and constant presence of this neurotransmitter. More energy may be required to rectify this situation than to maintain it, and so the muscle fiber remains short, thereby increasing tension. This leads to a reduction in oxygen and increased anaerobic metabolism, resulting in abnormal depolarization of the post-junctional membrane of the motor endplates.

Resultant ischemia develops and creates an oxygen/nutrient deficit, accompanied by a local energy crisis. Energy (ATP) is needed to remove the excessive calcium. ATP availability is decreased by the ensuing tissue tightness, which in turn restricts local blood supply. The persistent high calcium levels maintain ACh release. A vicious cycle results.

ACh transmission causes the actin and myosin elements of myofibrils to glide into a shortened position, leading to the formation of contractures (involuntary, without action potential). More energy is required for removing excessive calcium than for sustaining a contracture, and so the contracture remains.

Contractures are sustained by the chemistry at the innervation site, not by action potentials; they are to be differentiated from contractions (voluntary with action potentials) and spasms (involuntary with action potentials). The actin/myosin filaments glide into a fully shortened position (a weakened state) in the immediate area around the motor endplate (positioned at the center of the fiber). As the sarcomeres shorten, a contracture "nodule" forms—a palpable characteristic of a trigger point. The remainder of the sarcomeres on either side of this nodule within that fiber are lengthened, thereby creating a palpable taut band—another common trigger point characteristic. Other characteristics are spot tenderness of a nodule in the taut band, and the patient's recognition of pain or sensation when pressure is applied to the tender nodule.

Additionally, there may be:

1. Visual/tactile/autonomic evidence of local twitch response (LTR).
2. Pain or altered sensation in the target zone associated with that trigger point when provoked.
3. An EMG demonstration of spontaneous electrical activity (SEA) in the nidus (nucleus) of the trigger point.
4. A painful limit to full stretch and reduced range of motion.
5. A positive test of weakness of the muscle housing the trigger point.
6. Changes in cutaneous humidity (dry or moist), temperature (cool or hot), or texture (rough).
7. A "jump sign" or exclamation by the patient because of extreme tenderness of palpated tissues.

Myofascial trigger points are often associated with the feeling of ropy bands beneath the palpating fingers. Locating and identifying these bands requires excellent palpation skills and knowledge of the cardinal signs. Placing the muscle in a lengthened position may exaggerate the ropy bands and should make them more noticeable to "listening" fingers. Contraction knots can be small or large, depending on a variety of factors, such as the number of myofascial trigger points making up the contraction knots, the tissue consistencies, and the amount of fluid infiltration involved.

When a muscle is burdened with multiple myofascial trigger points, there is pain when that muscle is either lengthened or the myofascial trigger point is compressed. Pain occurs at the end range of motion (EROM) of the muscle in question, restricting ease of movement. The myofascial trigger point, in each muscle, causes a recognizable referral pattern. Sometimes those patterns are in the locality of the myofascial trigger points, but they may also cover several muscles. The patterns may not even include the muscle that holds the myofascial trigger points at all, as myofascial trigger points can *refer* pain and can alter sensations. Imagine having a constant itch you cannot scratch, ever. Imagine a noise in your ear that will not go away, ever—you have to find the myofascial trigger points that cause the symptoms and treat them. Myofascial trigger points mimic everything.

Each myofascial trigger point has its own recognizable pattern—a portrait of pain or changes in sensations. Simons, Travell, and Simons (1999) highlighted the difference between what are known as "active" myofascial trigger points and "latent" myofascial trigger points. Pain and changes in sensations from active myofascial trigger points are recognized by the patient as "their pain." Latent myofascial trigger points, on the other hand, cause pain that is not necessarily recognized by the patient but may be contributing to the patient's problems. Latent and active myofascial trigger points provoke motor dysfunction and impaired muscle activation patterns (Lucas et al. 2004, 2009), weakness, and muscle imbalances. It is vital to appreciate that latent myofascial trigger points can develop into active myofascial trigger points. The pain patterns in this book do *not* have an "X" to "mark the spot" of the myofascial trigger point, as may be found in other texts and books. It is important for everyone to understand that myofascial trigger points can occur *anywhere* in *any* muscle fiber.

Dry needling is an effective treatment for chronic pain of neuropathic origin and has been demonstrated to have very few side effects. This technique is unequalled in eliminating neuromuscular dysfunction of myofascial trigger point origin that results in pain, functional adaptations, and neuromuscular deficits.

Uniquely, this text provides all suitably qualified therapists with safe, effective, and appropriate clinical applications as part of a multidisciplinary approach, since only rarely can a single modality offer the intervention required for therapeutic success. Dry needling alone as a means of treating local myofascial trigger point pathology will almost certainly fall short of what is required for a complete rehabilitation.

If a muscle is sensitive and shortened or has active myofascial trigger points within it, the patient may feel a combination of sensations and pain. On compression, or needling, the patient can often feel a reproduction of "their" pain (active trigger point). This is a helpful diagnostic indicator for the practitioner when attempting to identify the true cause of the patient's symptoms.

A New Hypothesis

I wish to offer a new hypothesis while making a stark differentiation between myofascial trigger points and muscle spasm. A muscle spasm requires neural input (monosynaptic reflex arc) and ATP. Wearing my clinical anatomist's hat, I appreciate the fact that, on death, muscles take on a contracted state we call *rigor mortis* (Latin *rigor* means "stiffness," and *mortis* means "of death"). My hypothesis is that some, if not all, myofascial trigger points are a rigor contraction—an electromagnetic entity requiring no neural input and no need for ATP. This is an issue arising at the microscopic level, where the sarcomeres involved are only doing what they have evolved to be excellent at doing—contracting. To differentiate this "out of the normal" type of contraction, we refer to it as a "contracture." The all-or-none principle would have all the sarcomeres contracting, or none contracting.

In the case of a myofascial trigger point, approximately 100 sarcomeres are in a state of contracture within a cluster of myofascial trigger points. Higher up than the microscopic level, at the gross level, what is occurring would require manual therapies, such as positional release, soft tissue release, or other. Regarding the microscopic level, I propose that the needle only has to come into the proximity of the myofascial trigger point to elicit a change in polarization, causing a twitch response. Research to confirm or disprove this hypothesis is called for. Once normal electromagnetic activity has been restored, tensional and compressional forces also return to normal, and regular cellular activity can resume.

Standards and Guidelines in Myofascial Trigger Point Dry Needling

Anatomical Excellence

The therapist must pay scrupulous attention to anatomical detail. Before inserting the needle, the therapist is advised to check and recheck anatomical landmarks to ensure that they will avoid neural (or other) structures that could suffer insult. The use of needles is an invasive technique that carries a risk of infection to both the patient and the therapist. While it is important that therapists follow local, state, national, or international best practice, some additional standards and guidelines are presented in this chapter.

General Standards and Guidelines—Pre-treatment

- Ensure you have your patient's signed consent before dry needling.
- Hands must be properly washed, with soap and lukewarm water, and be clean before beginning every treatment.
- Nails should be smooth and short.
- Single-use disposable paper towels are recommended.

- Single-use gloves should always be worn by the therapist when handling a needle and for applied compression of the needled area following removal of the needle.
- The skin over which the treatment will be applied should be cleaned; however, in accordance with the WHO recommendations, it need not be disinfected.
- Single-use needles contained in delivery tubes are essential and must be used before their expiry date (check packaging for details).
- Needle thickness varies and should reflect the patient's needs and the anatomical location of the treatment, e.g., hands and face versus thigh.
- Avoid touching the needle shaft.
- Therapists should follow national guidelines and standards provided by a competent authority within their own geographical location or follow international best practice if such standards are not locally in place.
- Therapists must carry out a full medical health screening in advance of any treatment to ensure the patient's suitability

for the procedure, and to provide a comprehensive description of the procedure, including all potential risks.

- Target the four most significant symptoms. Identify all the known and suspected perpetuating factors: control the known ones and investigate the suspected ones. Include tests (such as a sleep study), exercise regimens (including correct breathing technique), and dietary changes.
- Therapists providing dry needling should also be qualified in emergency first aid (first responder), and, although not essential, I recommend courses that include defibrillation.

General Standards and Guidelines—Post-treatment

- Single-use needles should be disposed of in a sharps container, following local disposal regulations for blood-contaminated needles.
- Any disposables—such as cotton wipes or similar—should be disposed of in an appropriate manner.
- Allow the adult patient appropriate time on the treatment table before they return to standing.
- If myofascial trigger point dry needling causes the eyes to water post-treatment, advise your patient to allow appropriate time before driving.
- Encourage your patient to take it easy over the following day or so, and to avoid repetitious or stressful movements. The patient will require energy to accommodate and facilitate change post-treatment. Dry needling can also cause

some muscle soreness, similar to delayed onset muscle soreness, which can last from one to three days. Therapists should ensure that their patients are aware of this.

- Patients should avoid very cold (ice) applications, hot baths or showers, saunas, or steam rooms for a number of days following treatment.
- Cool water is the post-treatment of choice.

General Standards and Guidelines—During Treatment

- Take appropriate steps to ensure patient comfort.
- To ensure the best possible treatment outcomes, it is advisable to avoid treating too many muscles in a single treatment: it is recommended to limit treatment to between three and five muscles in any one treatment. Keep in mind, however, that this could constitute many hundreds of myofascial trigger points. The patient must have the capacity to facilitate changes as a result of the treatment. Less in this case is more. Practitioners can complement the treatment with other non-invasive modalities.
- The uncovered hand and fingers can be used to locate the myofascial trigger point and to identify key anatomical landmarks; however, to ensure the safe application of this technique, gloves must be worn when handling or using the needle or whenever there is a risk of contamination.
- On removal of the needle, ischemic pressure should be applied for a suitable length of time to minimize any blood loss.

- Any blood on the skin should be wiped with an alcohol swab, which should then be appropriately discarded.
- Regular communication with the patient is advised during the treatment, ensuring feedback and information is received from the patient.
- Look for non-verbal signs, such as facial expression, breath holding, and clenching.
- Treatment is generally not recommended with the patient in the seated position (because of the risk of fainting).

Wearing Gloves

While writing this book I received feedback regarding the recommendation that gloves should be worn when carrying out dry needling. The reviewer stated: "It is practically impossible to perform dry needling while wearing gloves." Wearing gloves can bring issues of reduced kinesthetic awareness and awkwardness in handling the needles. However, while opinions may differ, my responsibility as an author is to provide the safest recommendations to the therapist. I realize, of course, that palpation awareness and tactile feedback will be somewhat reduced with the wearing of latex or similar gloves.

The main reason for the use of gloves is that when a needle is withdrawn from a muscle, the most common side effect is bleeding. Whenever there is a possibility that the therapist's skin could come into contact with the patient's blood, care must be taken to provide a barrier and appropriate protection for the therapist.

Of secondary benefit is the fact that gloves provide an additional (albeit minimal) layer of "skin" to the therapist, and therefore the risk of needle stick is further reduced (if only fractionally). Gloves provide such protection and therefore must be recommended. In fact, it is worth noting that a number of insurance companies will not provide cover unless the therapist demonstrates that they wear gloves during the dry needling application.

Risks and Cautions in Myofascial Trigger Point Dry Needling

1. Some patients may experience an allergic reaction to the needle.
2. Fainting (vasodepressor syncope). This reaction can be caused by emotional stress and a fear of pain.
3. Hematoma (muscle bruising). Appropriate post-needling ischemic pressure will in general significantly reduce the possibility of developing a hematoma.
4. Prosthetic implants and implanted devices must be declared since dry needling is contraindicated for such patients because of the risk of infection.
5. Nerve damage/injury or nerve block is rare but can occur.
6. Damage to a vein or artery is rare but can occur.
7. Insult to the spinal cord or brain is rare but can occur.
8. Inserting a needle into any of the internal viscera or through a fenestrated bone (a bone with small holes in it) is rare but can occur.
9. When infection is present, dry needling must be avoided.

10. Increased muscle spasm, increased pain, and muscular edema can occur.

Myofascial trigger point dry needling will not be suitable for all adult patients. If, for any reason, a patient is not able to give consent to the procedure, or if they seem confused in any way, then dry needling must not be applied. Check the patient's skin for signs of swelling or possible lymphedema, as the application of dry needling could increase the risk of infection. In fact, there may be days when patients who normally receive this treatment may be better advised to avoid it. Care should be taken to discuss the suitability of this technique with each patient, considering each case individually and on its own merits.

Explaining to patients in advance of the application the entire procedure and what to expect during treatment and post-treatment will help to ensure that your patients are well informed. Needles identical to those used in this unique application have been used daily for many years by thousands of therapists across the world. In appropriately qualified hands, needling is a very safe technique.

Contraindications to Myofascial Trigger Point Dry Needling

1. Open wounds or broken skin should be avoided.
2. Malignancies. Should a patient state they have a malignancy, their GP or specialist must give written permission before any treatment can be given.
3. Aneurysm.

4. Hematomas. These should never be pressed, massaged, or stretched.
5. Arteriosclerosis. Because of the risk of blood clot formation, a GP's or medical specialist's approval must be given in writing. Information regarding all medications should be provided.
6. Osteoporosis. This is particularly serious if using dry needling techniques because of the risk posed by fenestrations (e.g., small holes in the scapula, through which the needle could pass and contact the lungs if care is not taken).

Ruling Out Visceral Pain—"When in Doubt, Refer"

Visceral pain has a temporal evolution, and in its early stages can be insidious and difficult to identify. Because of the low density of sensory innervation of viscera, and the extensive divergence of visceral input within the central nervous system (CNS), what is called "true" visceral pain is a vague, diffuse, and poorly defined sensation, regardless of the specific internal organ of origin. This type of pain is usually perceived in the midline, at the level of the lower sternum or upper abdomen. Whether it originates from the heart, esophagus, stomach, duodenum, gallbladder, or pancreas, visceral pain in the early phase is perceived in this same general area.

Additional stimuli, such as local compression, applied to this area fail to worsen the pain. True visceral pain can easily be overlooked, partly because the patient cannot clearly describe the pain. It is often described as a vague sense of discomfort, malaise, or oppression. The pain is typically associated with marked autonomic phenomena, such as pallor, profuse sweating, nausea, vomiting, changes in blood pressure and heart rate, gastrointestinal disturbances (e.g., diarrhea), and changes in body temperature. Strong emotional reactions are commonly present, including anxiety, anguish, and sometimes even a sense of impending death. Visceral pathology may occasionally manifest principally through vegetative and emotional reactions, with minimal pain and discomfort. A typical example is painless myocardial infarction, which may produce a sense of gastric fullness, heaviness, pressure, squeezing, or choking.

In the early stages, as a general rule, the intensity of visceral pain bears no relationship to the extent of the internal injury. Visceral pain should always be suspected when your patient presents with vague midline sensations of malaise. This is even further compounded when the patient is elderly.

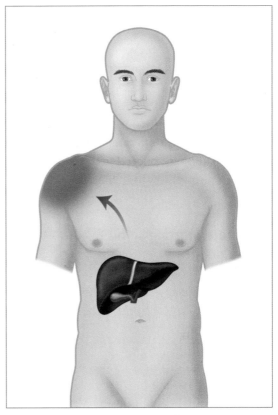

Figure 2.1. Potential referral site from liver pathology.

As visceral pain continues to progress (over a few minutes to several hours), it may refer to dermatomes whose innervations enter the spinal cord at the same level as the visceral organ involved. This can be misinterpreted by the brain as joint, muscular, or nerve pain manifesting itself as sharp, localized, deep somatic pain. For example, liver pathology can lead to referred pain in the upper right shoulder (figure 2.1). Peripheral nerve pathology, such as irritation of the C7–8 spinal nerves, presents as pain in the fourth and fifth digits (ulnar nerve). This type of pain can be accompanied by hyperalgesia (increased sensitivity, pain on light stimulation) or hypoalgesia (decreased sensitivity, numbness).

Detailed questioning of a patient is necessary to clarify their suitability for the treatment and their level of discomfort. During this assessment, the therapist must determine the characteristics of the pain, the pathways of pain radiation or referral, and the form and dependency of the pain on active, active resisted, or passive movements. Feedback from the patient concerning neurological signs, skin sensitivity, pain, and referral, as well as other symptoms, including heat, cold, tingling, itch, and mood swings, are all vital ammunition in the war on pain. This information will ensure that the patient is referred to the appropriate medical practitioner if warranted. If you are in any doubt at all, refer the patient to their health care provider, who will respect you for your professional approach and concern for the patient's health and wellbeing.

Once your patient returns to you, they must supply a letter from their health care provider stating that pathology is not suspected and has been ruled out. As time can be such a crucial factor in pathology, referral without delay is always in the patient's best interests.

Before Starting—The Ten-Point Guidelines

The following safety-first guidelines are applicable for both the post-screening and pre-needling stages:

1. Check your anatomical landmarks. Check again and be sure.
2. Use your palpation skills: a) identify autonomic responses, and b) identify the myofascial trigger point by digital application.
3. Put on your protective gloves.
4. Check your anatomical landmarks once again, and then place the needle within the delivery tube over the area to be treated. Release the needle.
5. Insert the needle with a firm fast "tap" (observe for any reaction).
6. Treat the myofascial trigger point with straight in-and-out motions.
7. Allow the patient to control the situation: encourage them to breathe slowly through the nose on the inhale and with pursed lips on the exhale.
8. Deactivate all the myofascial trigger points in any one muscle (treat the muscles which are most superior and medial first) and

avoid treating more than five muscles in any one treatment.
9. After removing the needle, apply ischemic pressure to the tissue and return the needle backward (handle first) into the delivery tube.
10. Discard all used needles and contaminated items safely in the sharps container or other appropriate waste disposal unit, which should be close to hand.

A Few Words About Dietary Influences

Adequate quantities of minerals and vitamins are essential for healthy muscles and tissues. Many patients presenting with chronic pain are found to be deficient in a number of vitamins and minerals. Vitamins B_1, B_6, and B_{12}, along with vitamin C and folic acid, are important in the war on pain; the minerals calcium, magnesium, iron, and potassium are critically important.

All too often, people are confused as to why they are deficient in these important minerals and vitamins, because they will report that they eat well and have normal dietary habits compared with other family members. The problem may not be their diet but rather their personal health choices, such as smoking and drinking alcohol or caffeine. Smoking, for example, annihilates vitamin C, while oral contraceptives affect vitamin B_6 levels. Antacid medication can leave many individuals with the symptoms of chronic fatigue; even writing their signature becomes an effort.

Patients with vitamin and/or mineral deficiencies may report feeling unusually cold, bouts of diarrhea, restless leg syndrome, headaches, disturbed sleep, and trigger point pain. Other symptoms include feeling fatigued, muscle cramping, and depression. Metabolic disorders should be ruled out, particularly thyroid problems and hypoglycemia. Referral of patients with vitamin/mineral deficiencies is recommended.

Needle Application

After removing the delivery tube from its packaging, place the delivery tube against the skin and release the needle. Quickly tap the needle into the tissue over the target muscle, ensuring that the needle is securely inserted just beneath the skin. Remove the delivery

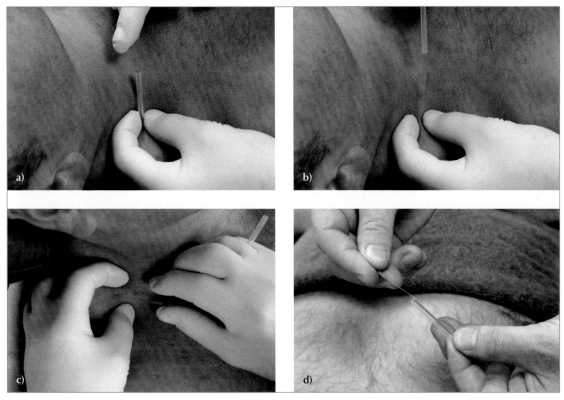

Figure 2.2. Procedure. (a) After removing the delivery tube from its packaging, place the delivery tube against the skin and release the needle. Quickly tap the needle into the tissue over the target muscle, ensuring that the needle is securely inserted just beneath the skin. (b) Remove the delivery tube. (c) Place the delivery tube between your fourth and fifth fingers. Use straight in-and-out motions to direct the needle to its target. Elicit a twitch response and proceed to eliminate all twitch responses. If the patient experiences burning or undue pain, immediately withdraw the needle and reposition the needle when the patient is ready and relaxed. Never bend the needle, especially when inserted, and avoid inserting the needle completely, while keeping a firm grip on the needle handle. (d) Returning the needle to the tube via the opposite end to the <u>handle must be avoided,</u> as this significantly increases the risk to the therapist of a needle stick. In other words, needles must be returned to the delivery tubes <u>handle first.</u> Wearing gloves during the needling application is recommended.

tube and place it between your fingers. Use straight in-and-out motions to direct the needle to its target.

Elicit a twitch response and proceed to eliminate all twitch responses. If the patient experiences burning or undue pain, immediately withdraw the needle and reposition the needle when the patient is ready and relaxed. *Never* bend the needle, especially when inserted, and avoid inserting the needle completely, while keeping a firm grip on the needle handle.

Returning the needle to the tube via the opposite end to the handle *must be avoided*, as this significantly increases the risk to the therapist of a needle stick. In other words, needles must be returned to the delivery tubes *handle first*. Wearing gloves during the needling application is recommended.

Direct the Needle with Straight In-and-Out Motion

Remember, *never* try to bend the needle or change needle direction when it is already in the muscle.

Health and Safety Considerations

Who (and What) Should Not Receive Dry Needling?

- Avoid dry needling patients who are clinically obese or whose body fat is below a safe level. Likewise, avoid needling patients who are intoxicated or fatigued, have an acute medical condition (such as epilepsy), or are pregnant. Patients with a needle phobia, or those who are unwilling, confused, or unable to give consent, should not receive myofascial trigger point dry needling.
- Nerves, blood vessels, and areas of lymphedema should be avoided. Patients who have bleeding tendencies or problems with blood clotting, or those taking blood-thinning (anticoagulant) medication, should avoid dry needling unless they are under the strict guidance of a medical practitioner. Patients with compromised immune systems are more susceptible to infection, as are patients with vascular disease and artificial joints and implants; in such cases, seek medical advice.
- Patients with pacemakers should avoid dry needling.
- Cancer patients should not receive dry needling, while for those with epilepsy more caution is required because of their low tolerance to strong sensory stimulation.
- Dry needling should be avoided when there is knowledge or evidence of infection, ulcers, osteoporosis, trauma/open wounds, aneurysm, or malignancy.
- Patients with psychological disorders may not be potential candidates for dry needling: emotional stress and anxiety may render dry needling unsafe. In such cases, medical advice must be sought.

Informing Patients

Dry needling is an invasive technique: needles break the skin and are placed either superficially or deep in the tissues, which brings with it associated risks. Your responsibility as a therapist is to clearly inform your patients of the risks involved and receive their written permission before placing a needle in their body. Patients must also be informed about possible side effects and needle effects, both immediate and longer term. Patients have the right to refuse a treatment or to cease a treatment at any time.

Patient Responsibilities

Each adult patient has the responsibility to provide information accurately and honestly to the therapist. Patients should notify therapists about any conditions that they have which can be transferred by blood, or about conditions that require blood anticoagulants or that may be adversely affected by needle punctures.

Pain During Needle Insertion

Pain experienced during insertion of the needle will most likely be due to a therapist's heavy-handed technique or awkwardness, usually because of lack of experience. Needle thickness and length must be appropriate to the target muscles or body part; for example, the hands, feet, and face are extremely sensitive and require a fine needle gauge. A blunt or hooked needle must never be used and will naturally cause the patient unnecessary pain. Pain may also occur in highly sensitive patients.

In most cases, skillful insertion of the needle through the skin with the appropriate level of controlled speed results in painless penetration of the deeper tissues. Participation in a formal course of studies under the watchful eye of a qualified and properly experienced tutor is essential. A qualified tutor will ensure that each therapist learns the correct technique while utilizing the optimum degree of force.

Avoiding Nerves and Blood Vessels

Nerves and blood vessels are literally everywhere in the human body, and so it is impossible to totally avoid one or the other. The largest blood vessels and nerves can be identified in several ways; to this end, knowledge of surface and gross anatomy is key (figure 2.3).

Major veins are often obvious to the eye, while deeper arteries can be pinpointed by palpation and therefore, as in the case of nerves, avoided. Blood vessels and nerves travel together as neurovascular bundles as they course through the septal divisions and the fascial conduits of the human body.

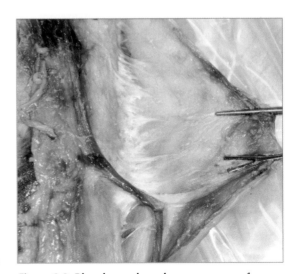

Figure 2.3. Blood vessels and nerves, many of which can be seen just below the skin, are avoided through excellent knowledge of anatomy. (Photograph: J. Sharkey 2008).

Guided Delivery Tube

This book recommends the use of a guided delivery tube to facilitate the smooth delivery and rapid penetration of the needle. The use of a needle guide tube allows the therapist to hold the needle steady over the skin while it is then tapped into place using the pad of the second digit (see the images showing needle insertion).

Pain After Needle Insertion

Several issues can arise while the needle is being inserted, resulting in the patient experiencing pain. Patients should be made aware of this in advance so that they are better prepared to deal with pain should it occur. The most obvious reason for pain when the needle is inserted is contact with nerve tissue; in this case, the needle should be returned to just below the surface of the skin and redirected. Needle grasping should also be considered: the needle may become interwoven and twist within the connected tissues, requiring a de-rotation of the needle or a gentle tapping on the top of the needle handle until the needle releases.

The therapist should look for any needle grasping and "tenting" (visible raising-up of the tissues and skin as a consequence of increased resistance to removing the needle) as the needle is removed. Work slowly with the patient and encourage controlled breathing, pursing the lips on exhaling. The therapist should never bend a needle: the needle motion is straight in and straight out.

Should the patient move during the application, this could affect the needle. Precautions should therefore be taken to minimize this possibility: the patient should be carefully positioned to provide the therapist with the greatest amount of control relating to unexpected reactive movement.

Post-needling Soreness

Soreness can occur within the first twenty-four hours following myofascial trigger point dry needling. This typically feels like delayed onset muscle soreness (what should be called "delayed onset myofascial soreness"), as if the muscle had been subjected to unaccustomed exercise or physical activity. Application of a cool pack or cold water to the area (ice is *not* recommended) should reduce any discomfort, which should normally not last more than a day. Applying contrast cold and heat therapy can also be useful, starting and ending with a cold application.

Central Sensitization and Control of Perpetuating Factors

Chronic pain syndromes display significant neuroplastic changes, altered neuron activity, and excitability and adaptations affecting pain matrix structures, specifically the spinal cord, thalamic nuclei, cortical areas, amygdala, and periaqueductal gray areas. In essence, central sensitization is characterized by an amplification of normal neurological activity (Giamberardino et al. 2011a).

Continuous bombardment of the dorsal horn by noxious afferent activity leads to a release of glutamate and substance P; this in turn leads to the activation of previously inactive synapses in the wide dynamic range (WDR), resulting in central sensitization. In normal circumstances, there is a balance between inhibitory and facilitatory neuronal activity in terms of pain management and control (Willard 2008). This results in "spinal segmental sensitization (SSS)"—a hyperactive state of the dorsal horn caused by constant noxious afferent bombardment, originating from damaged or sensitized tissues, e.g., myofascial trigger points or other soft tissue/connective tissue trauma, or visceral structures, such as a gallbladder that has become inflamed because

of gallstones (figure 3.1). A diagnosis of SSS includes observation of dermatomal allodynia, hyperalgesia, soft tissue pain/tenderness upon palpation, and myofascial trigger points (Giamberardino et al. 2011b).

Hypersensitivity initially occurs at the local segmental level. However, through the process of sensitization of adjacent spinal segments (spillover), a state of "wind-up" caused by "temporal sensory summation (TSS)"—an increased rate of nociceptive pulsing at the dorsal horn—facilitates widespread segmental sensitization, leading to body-wide peripheral pain. TSS is caused by increased C-fiber input at the dorsal horn and can maintain a state of hyperalgesia in chronic pain patients (Staud, 2011).

The stimuli that activate and sensitize the WDR neurons ascend the spinothalamic tract to reach the higher brain centers, where the thalamus and limbic systems are activated (anterior cingulate gyrus, insula, and amygdala). The limbic system is involved in modulating muscle pain, but it also modulates fear, anxiety, and distress. Therefore, increased activity in the limbic system, influencing

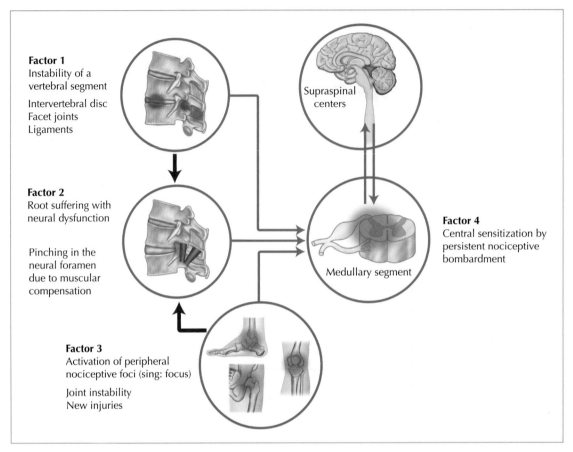

Factor 1
Instability of a
vertebral segment

Intervertebral disc
Facet joints
Ligaments

Factor 2
Root suffering with
neural dysfunction

Pinching in the
neural foramen
due to muscular
compensation

Factor 3
Activation of peripheral
nociceptive foci (sing: focus)

Joint instability
New injuries

Supraspinal
centers

Medullary segment

Factor 4
Central sensitization by
persistent nociceptive
bombardment

Figure 3.1. Spinal segmental sensitization.

the perpetuation of pain syndromes, can
contribute to the fear or emotional stress
associated with chronic pain syndromes
(Niddam et al. 2007).

The rostral ventral medulla (RVM), acting
as a relay point for descending activity from
the periaqueductal gray (PAG), contains a
number of "on" and "off" cells that can increase
or decrease levels of pain. In the acute phase
of injury, the "on" cells provide a protective
mechanism—significant pain is evoked,
thereby preventing undue movement/activity
that might cause more damage. In chronic
pain mechanisms, "on" cells remain active, and
there appears to be an "on" cell dominance,

rather than a balance of "on" and "off" cells that
would maintain a balance between facilitation
and inhibition (Willard 2008). Additionally,
normal descending pain-inhibiting signals are
disrupted, leading to a further sensitization of
muscle tissue (Niddam et al. 2007).

Spinal Facilitation

Spinal facilitation is an increase in spinal
cord neuron activity as a result of noxious
peripheral nociceptor bombardment. In
normal circumstances, this noxious stimulus
is modulated by local mechanisms, or by
descending pathways from the cerebral

cortex and brainstem. Abnormal constant bombardment leads to cell apoptosis, wind-up, and segmental sensitization (Bishop, Beneciuk, and George 2011). As a consequence, the dorsal, ventral, and lateral horn circuits in the spinal cord may become more readily activated by lower intensity stimuli.

Spinal facilitation is characterized by, 1) increased ventral horn output, which results in increased muscle tone (corresponding to the segmental level); 2) increased lateral horn output, which increases nociceptive activity (reflex mechanisms); and 3) increased dorsal horn activity, resulting in an increase in the production of neuropeptides, which can increase inflammatory activity in the affected tissues. The result is increased hyperalgesia, local tissue tenderness, and spillover, which affect adjacent spinal segments (Camanho, Imamura, and Arendt-Nielsen 2011).

Note

Too often doctors and therapists fail to consider the role of myofascial trigger points in chronic pain patients. They therefore fail to treat what may be, at least, a significant underlying perpetuating factor.

Many therapists deactivate myofascial trigger points as they find them, without giving due consideration to the mechanisms that caused them. In such cases, patients enjoy temporary relief but continue to have recurring pain issues that never fully resolve. Therapists can identify symptoms of spinal segmental sensitization and spinal facilitation by evaluating presenting symptoms of allodynia, hyperalgesia, pain pressure sensitivity, and motor and sensory

responses (reflex tests, dermatome assessment, and local muscle endurance assessment). Continuous nociceptive bombardment of the spinal cord leads to increased peripheral sensitivity and a state of central sensitization (Shah and Gilliams 2008).

Active and latent myofascial trigger points are found in the tissues of both symptomatic and asymptomatic individuals. Dorsal horn neurons may manifest neuroplastic changes as a result of nociceptive bombardment if left unresolved.

Cortical changes amplify the pain state, creating a pain cycle that may be difficult to break, as in the case of chronic pain conditions such as fibromyalgia, chronic fatigue syndrome, and myalgic encephalomyelitis (Camanho, Imamura, and Arendt-Nielsen 2011). Many people do not appreciate that stress is a normal part of living. It is how our body deals with stress and how we cope and deal with our sensory impressions, and how they stack up against our internal view of our world, that results in distress or eustress. This is part of our fight or flight system, or our ability to confront, avoid, or submit. Failure to resolve a stressful situation by one of these means results in high sympathetic tone, increased cortisol production, increased resting muscle tone, and the possible formation of myofascial trigger points. Myofascial trigger points are more likely to develop in tissue which has neurological deficits that have been caused by compression, tension, disc dysfunction, facet joint dysfunction, vascular compression, metabolic stress, biomechanical stress, postural stress, etc.

When muscles develop myofascial trigger points, they remain tight, causing local compression of vascular, neurological, and joint/biomechanical structures, thereby hampering the normal function of that tissue. All tissues distal to the nerve involved will likely be affected. Dry needling can release the muscle tension to resume normal function, with improved neurological conduction and vascularity. Dry needling should be supported by other appropriate soft tissue manipulation modalities and suitable physical activity.

Keys to Symptom Management

The following ten key aspects should be considered when treating myofascial trigger points:

1. Differentiate the myofascial trigger points from pain points by using the cardinal signs, which must include palpable nodule and taught band, jump sign, twitch response, painful EROM, referred pain, and autonomic responses.
2. Treat the myofascial trigger points that are most superior and medial first.
3. The deltoid seldom develops its own active myofascial trigger points. Instead, most are "baby" or "satellite" myofascial trigger points; therefore, treat associated muscles within the functional units of the deltoid first.
4. The upper trapezius is the "grand central station" of myofascial trigger points and is a major contributor to neck, shoulder, upper back, and head pain.
5. Active myofascial trigger points, when irritated by a competent therapist, will result in referred pain or changes in sensation that the patient recognizes.

6. Latent myofascial trigger points generally result in pain or change in sensations that the patient does not recognize. These myofascial trigger points may be contributing to, but are not the true source of, a patient's problem.
7. Myofascial trigger points can form in any muscle fiber (Sharkey 2008) and not just in the center of a muscle, or where the "X" marks the spot (which is misleading) on so many myofascial trigger point charts. Identify and remove/change the perpetuating factor(s).
8. Excellent palpation skills are necessary for locating myofascial trigger points.
9. Upper or lower limb tension tests should be administered to rule out nerve insults, including compression and/or inflammation.
10. Any patient suffering from unresolved pain or changes in sensations should have the possibility of myofascial trigger point involvement ruled out as a primary or secondary cause or contributor.

Initiating, Aggravating, and Perpetuating Factors

Anything that perpetuates a myofascial trigger point is called a "perpetuating factor." What initially activates a myofascial trigger point may be different from what aggravates (worsens) or perpetuates (maintains) it, but they are all commonly called perpetuating factors. The key to controlling any symptom is the control of as many perpetuating factors as possible.

An appropriate medical history will indicate whether pain patterns are stable or evolving. Chronic myofascial pain (CMP) is not progressive. The development of satellite myofascial trigger points that worsen symptoms, and the appearance of new symptoms, are indicators that there are perpetuating factors at play. To control symptoms, first identify and control perpetuating factors.

Controlling perpetuating factors is vital. Perpetuating factors include whatever impairs muscle function, such as anything that diminishes the cells' access to oxygen and nutrients, hampers the removal of cellular wastes, or adversely affects the metabolism of the neurotransmitter acetylcholine (ACh).

Anything that enhances the formation of myofascial trigger points is a perpetuating factor. For instance, anything that constricts the flow of blood to the area will lessen its supply of oxygen and nutrients, adding to the energy crisis. A perpetuating factor can be anything that increases energy demand (trauma, overwork), decreases energy supply (inadequate nutrition, insulin resistance), sensitizes the CNS (pain, noise), decreases oxygen supply (congestion), enhances the release of sensitizing substances (allergies, infections), or increases endplate noise (increased ACh release, reduced acetylcholinesterase).

Perpetuating Factor Types: A Long Short War

We are fighting a war on pain. The foot soldiers of the enemy are those perpetuating factors such as mechanical stressors, including paradoxical breathing, body disproportions,

myofascial or connective tissue abuse, and articular dysfunctions. Metabolic perpetuating factors include impairments to energy metabolism, and coexisting conditions, such as pain and a lack of restorative sleep. Environmental perpetuating factors include pollution, medications, trauma, and infections.

Psychological perpetuating factors are also an important area to investigate. The remedies for lifestyle perpetuating factors are often the least expensive but may be among the most difficult to maintain. To further complicate matters, perpetuating factors often have perpetuating factors of their own. Cognitive therapy and mindfulness can be useful interventions to help us change the way we, and our patients/ clients, think about and perceive pain.

Examples

"Paradoxical" (or "abdominal") breathing is a term used to describe an abnormal chest movement, with the patient's chest moving inward (or not moving at all) during inhalation rather than outward or forward. This means that your patient cannot take a functional breath and is most likely a shallow breather. Paradoxical breathing is a common perpetuating factor but is easy to check if a patient is presenting with this breath rhythm issue.

To assess for correct rhythm, place one hand on your patient's abdomen. As the patient breathes in, their abdomen should swell as the abdominal cavity extends after the lungs expand, and on breathing out, the patient's abdomen should come back in. When this occurs, it indicates that their respiratory muscles are healthy: the patient can move through their physiological range to accommodate the air required and expel residual air.

If the patient's chest is moving in as the breath comes in, and is moving out as the breath goes out, then this is paradoxical breathing. This inconsistent breathing includes mouth breathing, which is inefficient and shallow. Paradoxical breathing may indicate that your patient's body is not getting the oxygen it needs; it can occur temporarily during a time of congestion, such as a cold, and then may be maintained out of habit, or because myofascial trigger points have formed in the diaphragm or other respiratory muscles, thus inhibiting their function.

Training and awareness of proper breathing technique are important, but they are only part of the remedial process. Is adequate air coming in through the nose, or is there congestion? If so, why? Check into the possibility of allergies, low-grade sinusitis (sometimes caused by fungal infection), or other problems. A myofascial trigger point assessment is also needed, as myofascial trigger points can cause congestion, and their presence in respiratory muscles prevents these muscles from working properly. An assessment for myofascial trigger points includes accessory respiratory muscles, such as the scalenes and the serratus muscles.

Body Disproportion Examples

A structural leg inequality of 1/5 (as a fraction) in. (0.5 cm) can significantly tilt the body (figure 3.2). What is more common, however, especially in people with myofascial trigger

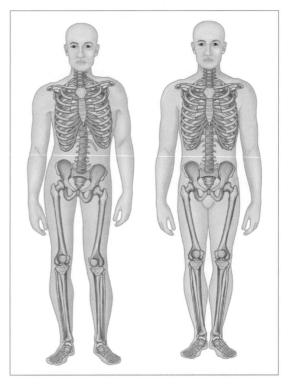

Figure 3.2. A structural leg inequality can significantly tilt the body.

points, is pelvic torsion, where one thigh is drawn higher into the pelvis, thereby creating a functionally short leg. In this case, if one adds a heel lift to the shorter leg, the problem is compounded and reinforced.

True leg length inequality is a clue to check the whole body for proportional shortness on that side and for compensation on the opposite side. When the horizontal core stabilizers, including the deep ligaments and tendons, are not at healthy lengths, a spiral compensating effect, "rotoscoliosis," can occur. This is a twisting of the tissues around the spinal column and can begin anywhere, resulting in torsion of the feet, ankles, knees, hips, and shoulders. One area rotates right and the other rotates left to compensate. The body seeks

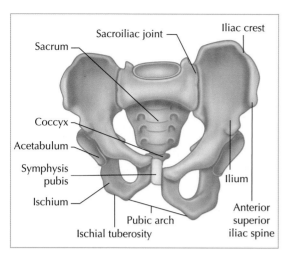

Figure 3.3. Hemipelvis.

harmony and balance, but this compensatory twisting can create functional hypermobility or restriction of numerous areas.

Another consideration is a one-sided small hemipelvis (figure 3.3). The right and left hemipelvis should match. When the hemipelvis is smaller on one side, if a patient is sitting on a flat surface, the upper curve of one hip is higher than the other.

Scoliosis and pelvic rotation can develop as other muscles struggle to compensate (figure 3.4). Quadratus lumborum is greatly affected by an asymmetrical hemipelvis, with the sternocleidomastoids and scalenes struggling to adjust to the overload from tilted thoracic muscles.

Muscle Abuse

Any postural habit that causes prolonged muscle fiber contraction, repetitive low-intensity overload, and muscle stress (such as high-intensity muscle contractions) can cause myofascial trigger points (Edwards

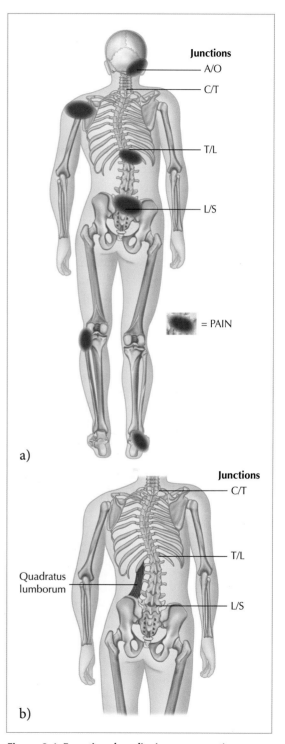

Figure 3.4. Functional scoliosis compensation.

2005). Posture affects respiration and can interact with vestibular dysfunction, thus compounding the symptoms (Yates, Billig, and Cotter 2002). Close attention must be paid to standing, sitting, work (figure 3.5) and sleeping postures (figure 3.6).

Any cervical pillow must fit the curvature of the neck to support it without stressing coexisting myofascial trigger points. The size and shape of the pillow may need changing as the neck and shoulders respond to treatment.

Once correct neuromuscular balance has been achieved, many bad posture habits can be identified and corrected; these include head-forward posture, bracing the arms on the knees, crossing the legs, side leaning, and crossing the arms to prop up weak muscles. Bad postural habits are often clues to the locations of myofascial trigger points or other perpetuating factors, such as facet pathology.

One of the most preventable types of perpetuating factor is inappropriate physical activity (exercise). It is almost impossible to strengthen muscles that have myofascial trigger points or that are inhibited without first resolving the hypertonic muscles. It is essential to initially restore neuromuscular balance between muscle units (targeting the short spastic muscle first) and then to encourage neuromuscular efficiency, rather than strength. Developing muscular strength of the inhibited muscle comes later in the sequence.

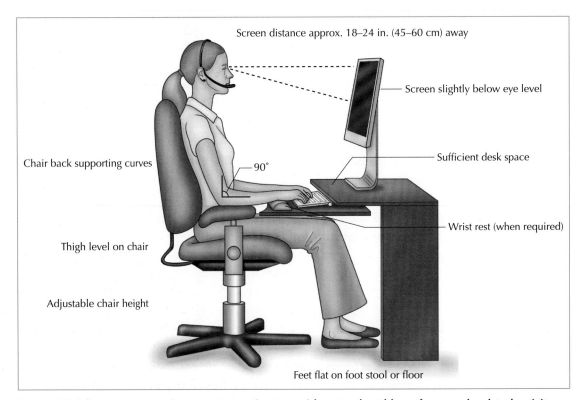

Screen distance approx. 18–24 in. (45–60 cm) away

Screen slightly below eye level

Chair back supporting curves

90°

Sufficient desk space

Thigh level on chair

Wrist rest (when required)

Adjustable chair height

Feet flat on foot stool or floor

Figure 3.5. Adopt an ergonomic computer station to avoid postural problems from work-related activity.

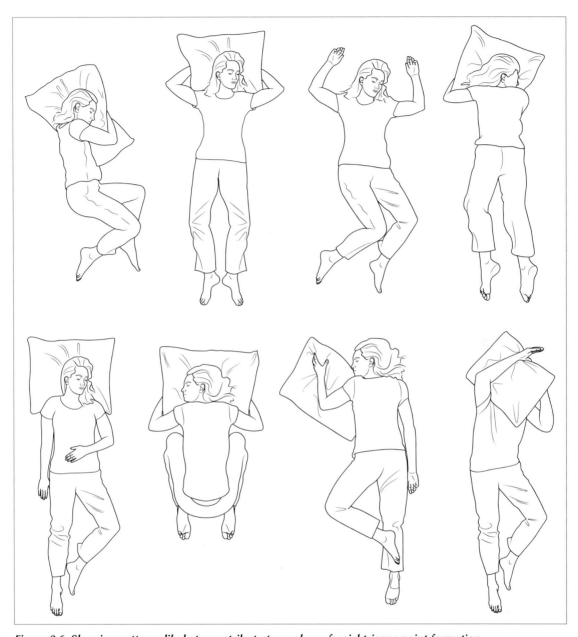

Figure 3.6. Sleeping patterns likely to contribute toward myofascial trigger point formation.

Articular Dysfunction

Joint dysfunction can interact with myofascial trigger points. Any mechanical stress affecting joint position can initiate the process of osteoarthritis (OA) (Solomon, Schnitzler, and Browett 1982). Treating myofascial trigger points improves neuromuscular function and coordination, and anything that improves neuromuscular function can prevent or slow the progression of OA (Loeser and Shakoor 2003).

Any arthritis treatment and prevention program needs to include the treatment of coexisting myofascial trigger points (Cummings 2003).

Myofascial trigger points can cause uneven contraction of muscles. An uneven contraction can cause or contribute to temporomandibular joint dysfunction (TMJD) and may cause bone misalignment (Koolstra and van Eijden 2005). Uneven muscle contraction may also be sufficient to cause jaw articular disc erosion (Liu et al. 2000).

Vertebrae and myofascial trigger points interact. Active myofascial trigger points are associated with neck vertebral-disc lesions (Hsueh et al. 1998). As surrounding soft tissues are unevenly contractured because of myofascial trigger points, vertebrae may shift slightly out of alignment; this misalignment irritates the intervertebral discs. Intervertebral disc adjustments, and their associated ligamentous attachment compensations, cause changes in the angular motion of the body, which further stresses the inferior and superior intervertebral discs of the cervical spine (Kumaresan, Yoganandan, and Pintar 1999).

Soft tissue is often neglected. Disc deterioration may further alter motion and muscle compensation, which can contribute to additional pathologies in facet joints, muscles, and ligaments, resulting in a chronic pain state (Brisby 2006). Disc deformities or bone spurs that show up on imaging, however, may not be the cause of pain. Surgery performed without soft tissue evaluations can result in failed back surgery (Dubousset 2003). Subsequent surgical scars, adhesions, and postsurgical tightening of soft tissue can cause added stress to adjacent vertebrae, leading to the formation of myofascial trigger points.

Treatment Options and Chronic Pain Management

A multidisciplinary approach is recommended when treating patients with chronic pain. Encouraging such patients to be actively involved in their own care is empowering and can also translate into therapeutic benefit. A combination of therapies seems to work best: treatment options can include (but are not limited to) myofascial release, frequency-specific microcurrent (McMakin 2011), positional release, galvanic stimulation, osteopathic therapy, craniosacral therapy, neuromuscular therapy, massage therapy, structural integration, medical exercise, and medical intervention.

Stretch and Spray—Active Cold Therapy Stretching

"Stretch and spray," also known as "active cold therapy stretching" (ACTS), is a technique that has been popularly used for more than twenty-five years with great effect. A vapocoolant spray is appropriately applied to the skin overlying the target muscle(s) while a stretch has been performed on the muscle(s). The technique requires the muscle(s) to be lengthened first to stimulate the muscle spindles before the spray is applied.

Stretch and spray is effective in the treatment of spastic tissue and is an excellent method for reducing or eliminating spastic activity. Modell et al. (1952) used a cold spray technique involving the application of spray, followed by an intense stretch. Travell purposely did not support the idea of "stretch and spray," as her recommendation was to apply the cold first as a distraction; the cold spray application was found to be useful, as it reduced pain and muscle tension. The stretch and spray technique is recommended primarily for treating spastic muscle or post-needling soreness.

Once the tissues are stretched, the cold spray is applied to deactivate the muscle spindles via the cooling effect on the skin surface. The spray follows the fasciculi arrangement and can be applied with three or four sweeps, from origin to insertion, without breaks between the sweeps. After the spray application, the area can be dried, and the target tissue brought to a shortened state for several seconds. The target tissues are then slowly returned to a new stretch barrier or resting length. This technique works best for spastic tissue but can be useful as a complement to myofascial trigger point needling, before or after its application.

Stretch and spray should only be carried out in a well-ventilated space, and steps should be taken to avoid inhaling the spray. The spray should be held at an appropriate distance from the skin to avoid freezing. Stretch and spray will not be suitable for all patients: avoid the procedure on persons with poor circulation or sensitive skin, and do not use spray or creams on open wounds or abraded skin. Only professionals qualified to do so should perform the stretch and spray (or similar) technique.

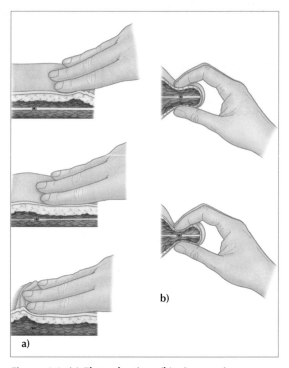

Figure 4.1. (a) Flat palpation, (b) pincer grip.

A Note on Palpation

Palpation is the act of touching with intent to diagnose or discover, and I freqently refer to two types of palpation throughout this book.

"Flat palpation" refers to the fingertips sliding across the muscle fibers. The skin is pushed to one side, and the finger is drawn across the muscle fibers. The process is then repeated with the skin pushed to the other side (figure 4.1a).

"Pincer grip" is where the belly of the muscle is gripped between the thumb and the forefinger, and the fibers are pressed between the fingers in a rolling manner (figure 4.1b).

Chronic Pain Management—Three Key Steps

There are three key steps to managing chronic pain:

1. Medical history/assessment
2. Special tests
3. Goal setting

Medical History/Assessment
A detailed medical history should be sought from every adult patient—details should include previous illness/injuries/allergies and history of all surgical interventions. In addition, a patient's current medication status provides important information in

Anaphylactic Reaction

Anaphylactic shock occurs due to the body's immune system reacting inappropriately in response to the presence of a substance that it perceives as a threat, and an anaphylactic reaction can occur when therapists use needles, sprays, creams, or oils. It is therefore essential that correct screening/medical history identifies those patients with a history of allergic reaction. Patients may fail to inform the therapist, or may simply get mixed up or forget, and so it is vitally important to take the appropriate precautions and have a first-responder plan of action in place in such an event.

An anaphylactic reaction results from the release of chemical substances, such as histamine. The release is initiated by the reaction between the allergic antibody (IgE) and the substance (allergen) causing the anaphylactic reaction. This mechanism is so sensitive that even minute quantities of the allergen can cause a reaction.

All therapists involved in myofascial trigger point therapy should be competent in the recognition and treatment of an anaphylactic episode. It is recommended that in all cases of allergic reaction a patient should make an appointment with their health care provider for appropriate advice.

determining if they are a suitable candidate for myofascial trigger point dry needling.

Patients frequently have more than one type of pain, as well as overlapping perpetuating factors. Careful pain assessment should include determining the mechanisms of pain. Document the pain location, changes in sensations, pain intensity, pain referral/radiation, quality/character of the pain, onset of pain (time and duration), functional ability, and perpetuating/relieving factors (see the photocopiable sample charts on pages 54 and 55 for patients to express their pain and provide location/referral information).

Psychological and social factors, depression or substance abuse, and allergies should also be taken into consideration. If there are any doubts or concerns regarding the root of the patient's pain, it is recommended to refer the patient to an appropriate primary medical care practitioner.

Special Tests

Special tests—including range of motion, thermal palpation, identification of autonomic responses, skin drags, skin rolling, or other orthopedic tests—are useful in locating the source of insult or the site of myofascial trigger points. Needle insertion that elicits a twitch response supports the diagnosis and presence of myofascial trigger points.

Goal Setting

Each treatment should have realistic short- and long-term therapeutic and functional goals. Simple achievable steps that offer motivation while providing encouragement to the patient are recommended. Medical exercise should be provided to support therapeutic interventions and should focus on physical activities that support daily function. An appropriate professional should also provide nutritional advice.

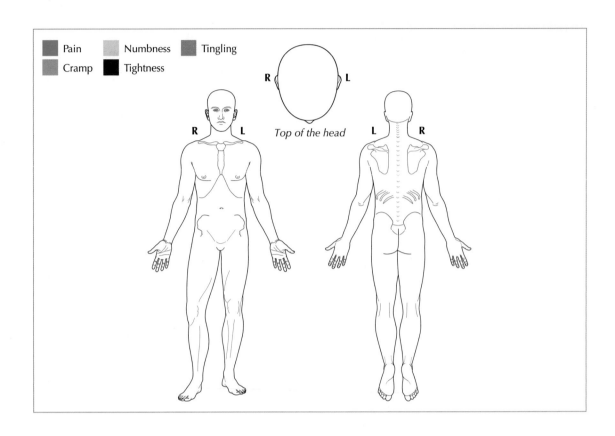

Patient: _____ Care provider: _____ Date: _____

Reason for visit: _____

Most distressing symptoms: _____

Additional patient comments (quality and nature of pain, aggravating factors, what has been tried

and results): _____

_____

Changes: _____

Needs (including prescriptions, therapies or tests): _____

_____

Action items (patient and care provider): _____

_____

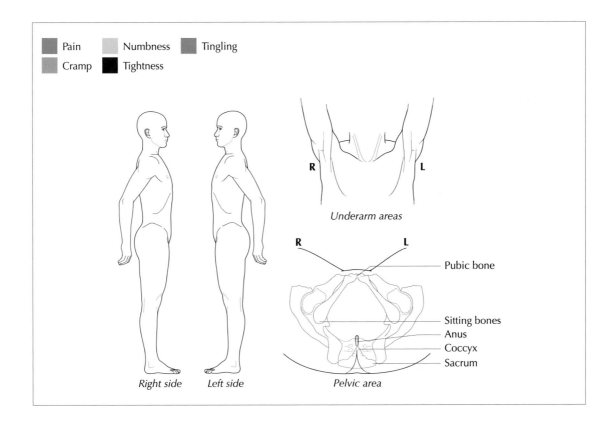

Pain   Numbness   Tingling
Cramp   Tightness

Underarm areas

R   L

Pubic bone

Sitting bones
Anus
Coccyx
Sacrum

Right side   *Left side*   *Pelvic area*

Patient: _____ Care provider: _____ Date: _____

Reason for visit: _____

Most distressing symptoms: _____

Additional patient comments (quality and nature of pain, aggravating factors, what has been tried

and results): _____

_____

Changes: _____

Needs (including prescriptions, therapies or tests): _____

_____

Action items (patient and care provider): _____

_____

Close monitoring will ensure that the various interventions are not overpowering the patient. Patients should be encouraged to keep a daily log to document their pain and sleep patterns. This log will provide a history of what aggravates their pain, when the onset of pain occurs, and when the pain is less or more intense, information which can often be revealing. Identifying the progression of the patient's pain will influence the choice of intervention and its intensity, as well as what outcome or rate of improvement or other should be expected. Improved sleep, coupled with improved respiratory function, can have a profound therapeutic effect. It is vital to take small steps, allowing a gradual return to homeostasis.

Having completed the key steps 1 to 3, the therapist is ready to develop a plan of therapeutic intervention. It is important to adopt an interdisciplinary team approach, with referral to, or involvement of, other specialists when there is a need for pharmacological, psychosocial, or physical activity (medical exercise specialist), or for any other management aspect outside your scope of practice.

A written plan of interventions and expected outcomes is an essential tool to ensure a comprehensive approach to treating a patient with chronic pain, and should address the person holistically, in all their complexity. Consideration should be given to physical and biological factors, psychological state and beliefs, and the family, social, and work environment.

Regular reassessment and appropriate goal adjustments are recommended.

Medications

While pain medications are useful and often essential, they should seldom be the sole focus of treatment in managing musculoskeletal pain. Pain medications should be used when needed to meet the overall goals of therapeutic intervention in line with medical advice.

Other treatment modalities need to be considered and the treatment modified on the basis of the effects of pain medications. Ensure that your patients follow medical advice.

PART II

MAJOR SKELETAL MUSCLES AND REFERRED PAIN PATTERNS

Muscles of the Face, Head, and Neck

OCCIPITOFRONTALIS

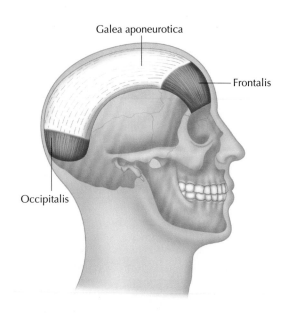

Galea aponeurotica

Frontalis

Occipitalis

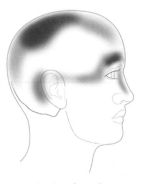

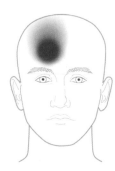

Occipitofrontalis

Frontalis

Latin, *occiput*, back of the head; *frons*, forehead, front of the head.

Origin
Occipital belly: Lateral two-thirds of the superior nuchal line of the occipital bone, and mastoid process of the temporal bone.
Frontal belly: Galea aponeurotica.

Insertion
Occipital belly: Galea aponeurotica.
Frontal belly: Fascia and skin above the eyes and nose.

Nerve
Facial VII nerve.

Action
Occipital belly: Moves the scalp backward. Assists the frontal belly to raise the eyebrows and wrinkle the forehead.
Frontal belly: Moves the scalp forward and wrinkles the skin of the forehead horizontally.

Kinetic Chain Comment

Occipitofrontalis is essentially two muscle bellies with a strong fascial connection between them, the "galea aponeurotica." Spasm in muscles such as the hamstrings (e.g., biceps femoris) or the plantar fascia can cause tightness through this area, ultimately causing tension in the head and neck, or headaches. Tension anywhere along the posterior back-line kinetic chain can lead to shortening of the galea aponeurotica, resulting in tension headaches and a hyperextended cervical spine. This can result in a posteriorly tilted pelvis to provide a level eye view when walking or running and is a recipe for myofascial trigger point formation.

Myofascial Trigger Point Comment

Pain is referred upward from the frontal belly over the forehead on the same side. The occipital belly can refer pain into the eyeball or behind the eye. Pain can travel down behind the ear and into the nose. Sensitivity to sound and light are reported, with a resulting increase in experienced pain. I have had patients who complained of severe pain "inside their head;" on investigation, myofascial trigger points in the occipital belly reproduced a recognizable pain.

Practitioner Guidelines

Patient positioning

Patient is supine to access frontal belly. For access to occipital belly, the head is rotated to the opposite side or the patient can be positioned prone.

Needle type

Use 0.25 to 0.30 mm × 30 mm needle.

Needling directions

Locate and secure the myofascial trigger point within the palpable taut band using flat palpation. Insert the needle and direct it tangentially into the myofascial trigger point. These are very slim/thin muscles and are best approached at a 45-degree angle.

Precautions

No special precautions.

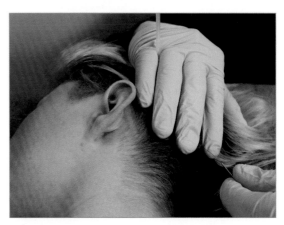

Occipital belly, side lying or supine, with head rotated to opposite side.

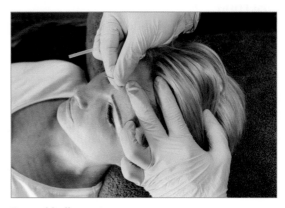

Frontal belly, supine.

TEMPORALIS

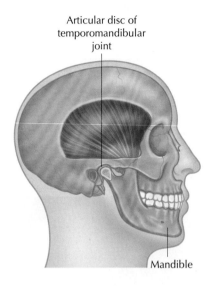

Articular disc of temporomandibular joint

Mandible

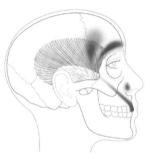

Lower front attachment TrP

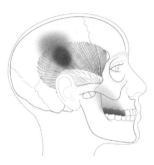

Lower rear attachment TrP (in front of ear area)

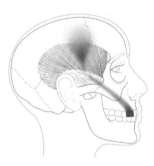

Lower center attachment TrP

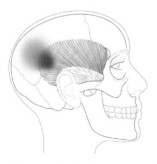

Central temporalis TrP (behind ear point)

Latin, *temporalis*, relating to the side of the head.

Origin

Deep surface of the temporal fascia, and the entire fossa. The floor of the fossa is made up of the zygomatic, frontal, parietal, sphenoid, and temporal bones.

Insertion

Medial/lateral apex and deep surfaces of the coronoid process of the mandible, and anterior border of the ramus of the mandible.

Nerve

Anterior and posterior deep temporal nerves from the trigeminal V nerve (mandibular division).

Action

Closes the jaw (elevates the mandible), assists side-to-side deviations of the mandible and clenching of the teeth. Pulls the ears up to create tension across the scalp.

Kinetic Chain Comment

Temporalis and masseter are synergists. An overdeveloped upper trapezius can be an overlooked contributor to problems associated with these muscles. A short temporalis leads to teeth clenching, which can damage the sensitive proprioceptive covering on the teeth. Temporal dysfunction can ensue, with loss of balance, vertigo, nausea, hearing difficulties, tinnitus, trigeminal neuralgia, and optical problems. The neck, face, and head muscles are as important to global muscle function as the core (lumbopelvic-hip complex). Habits such as chewing gum can cause repetitive stress and strain.

Myofascial Trigger Point Comment

One must appreciate the chain effect that an inhibited masseter could have on this muscle. Temporalis and masseter may develop myofascial trigger points in an effort to provide much-needed tension. A forward-head posture is most likely the evident posture. Pain passes upward and over the forehead on the ipsilateral side. Pain spills over just above the ear and into the nuchal line of the occiput. Temporalis should be considered in all headache patients.

Pain in the upper or lower teeth and gums is the most common pain pattern with this muscle. A deep pain has also been reported over the eyebrow and occasionally into the same side and back of the head. The treatment of other muscles on the basis of their pain referral patterns, if associated with this area, should also be carried out as part of the myokinetic chain.

Practitioner Guidelines

Patient positioning

Patient is supine or side lying, with the head rotated to the opposite side.

Needle type

Use 0.14 to 0.16 mm × 15 mm needle.

Needling directions

Locate and avoid the temporal pulse. Locate and secure the myofascial trigger point within the palpable taut band using flat palpation. Insert the needle and direct it toward the temporal fossa at a shallow angle.

Precautions

Palpate the temporal artery, which bifurcates into a frontal and a parietal portion. A shallow angle of needle insertion is recommended to avoid the deep anterior and posterior temporal arteries.

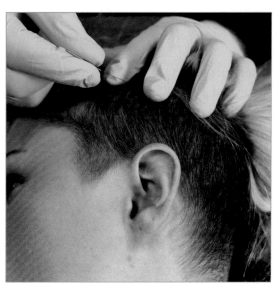

Temporalis with the head turned to the opposite side, supine.

MASSETER

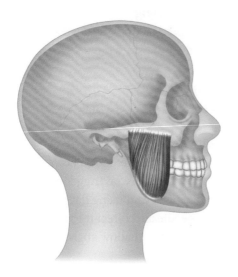

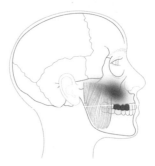

Superficial masseter upper attachment TrPs

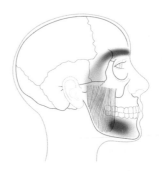

Superficial masseter lower attachment TrPs

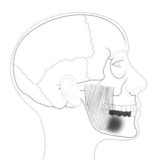

Superficial masseter central TrPs

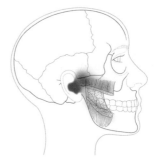

Deep masseter upper posterior TrPs

Greek, *maseter*, chewer.

Origin
Superficial portion: Zygomatic process of the maxilla, and anterior two-thirds of the zygomatic arch.
Deep portion: Surface of the zygomatic arch.

Insertion
Angle of the mandible, and outer surface of the ramus (superficial) and coronoid process of the mandible.

Nerve
Trigeminal V nerve (mandibular division).

Action
Closes the jaw. Elevation of the mandible and slight protraction of the jaw.

Kinetic Chain Comment

A forward-head posture places the mandible in a position that puts the masseter under undue stress. Antagonist muscles, such as the geniohyoid, omohyoid, and digastric, can all become spastic due to overtraining of the abdominal muscles using poor technique. This in turn may inhibit the masseter, with resulting myofascial trigger point formation to provide stiffness or tension within the muscle.

Changes in associated suboccipital muscles lead to changes in homeostasis of the head and face muscles. A change in the positioning of the temporomandibular joint will also affect the position of the cervical spine. Correct alignment of the temporomandibular joint requires treatment of the masseter and pterygoids at the local level, with attention to core efficiency at the global level.

Myofascial Trigger Point Comment

Masseter is a complex muscle, and pain is referred into the eyebrow, maxilla, mandible (anterior), and upper and lower molar teeth. Any person with a toothache will rightly go to a dentist. With no obvious pathology presenting, it is in the patient's best interests to rule out the possibility of referred pain from myofascial trigger points being at the root of the pain.

Other related sensations include hypersensitivity to pressure and temperature changes, e.g., during flights. Pain and changes in sensations can also refer into the temporomandibular joint and inner ear. Remember, it is not always about pain. Masseter myofascial trigger points are significant contributors to headaches.

Practitioner Guidelines

Patient positioning

Patient is supine or side lying, with the head rotated to the opposite side.

Needle type

Use 0.14 to 0.16 mm × 15 mm needle.

Needling directions

Locate and avoid needling the facial pulse and any visible vascular tissues around the area. Locate and secure the myofascial trigger point within the palpable taut band using flat palpation. Insert the needle and direct it either toward the mandible or toward the maxilla, with the mouth closed and the teeth surfaces touching.

Precautions

No special precautions.

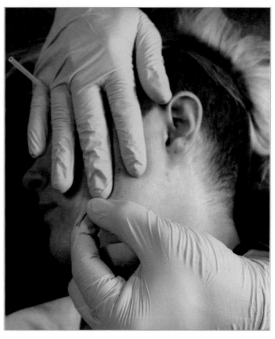

Masseter, supine with the head turned to the opposite side.

PTERYGOIDS

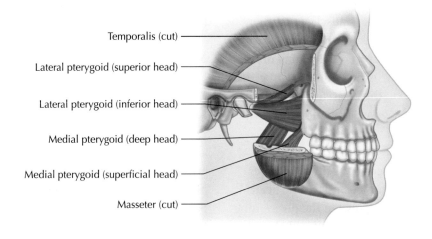

Temporalis (cut)

Lateral pterygoid (superior head)

Lateral pterygoid (inferior head)

Medial pterygoid (deep head)

Medial pterygoid (superficial head)

Masseter (cut)

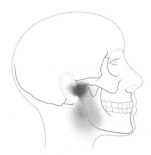

*Medial pterygoid
referred pain pattern*

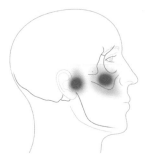

*Lateral pterygoid
referred pain pattern*

Greek, *pterygoeides*, wing-like. **Latin**, *medialis*, relating to the middle, *lateralis*, relating to the side.

Origin
Medial pterygoid
Deep head: Medial side of the lateral pterygoid plate, behind the upper teeth.
Superficial head: Maxillary tuberosity.
Lateral pterygoid
Superior head: Lateral surface of the greater wing of the sphenoid.

Inferior head: Lateral surface of the lateral pterygoid plate of the sphenoid.

Insertion
Medial pterygoid
Medial (fovea) angle of the mandible.
Lateral pterygoid
Capsule and articular disc of the temporomandibular joint, and neck of the mandible.

Nerve
Trigeminal V nerve (mandibular division).

Action
Medial pterygoid
Acts to elevate the mandible and close the jaw and helps the pterygoid lateralis in moving the jaw from side to side.
Lateral pterygoid
Opens the mouth, protrudes the mandible, and provides side-to-side movement.

Kinetic Chain Comment
Lower limb length inequalities cause mechanical stress which has been associated with myofascial trigger point formation in the neck muscles, especially sternocleidomastoid. Sternocleidomastoid in turn can be the site of mom or dad myofascial trigger points that form baby or satellite myofascial trigger points in the pterygoids. I do not encourage efforts to strengthen this muscle with resisted protrusion and static stretching; that, I believe, can offer short-term removal of symptoms but long-term reinforcement of the problems. A focus on removing myofascial trigger points is vital but must be followed by a program of appropriate physical activity involving full-body kinetic chain movement.

Myofascial Trigger Point Comment
Pain is referred deep into the temporomandibular joint and maxillary sinus. These myofascial trigger points are most often mistaken for arthritis or sinusitis. Pain has also been reported to be a causative factor in tinnitus. Pain can also be experienced in the tongue and the back of the mouth, with difficulty swallowing.

Practitioner Guidelines
Patient positioning
Patient is supine or side lying, with the head rotated to the opposite side.

Needle type
Use 0.14 to 0.16 mm × 15 mm needle.

Needling directions
Locate and avoid the facial pulse. Locate and secure the myofascial trigger point within the palpable taut band. Insert the needle while the patient keeps two fingers between their teeth to open the lower the angle of the mandible, allowing access to the muscle. If for any reason the patient pulls their fingers out of their mouth, there will be plenty of time for the therapist to quickly remove the needle before the mouth closes.

Precautions
Avoid needling the facial pulse and any visible vascular tissues around the area.

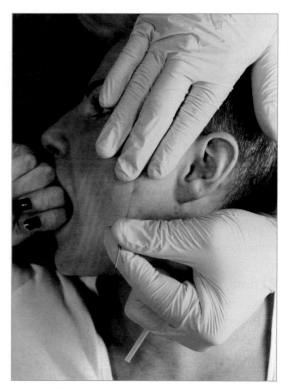

Pterygoids, supine with the head turned to the opposite side.

PLATYSMA

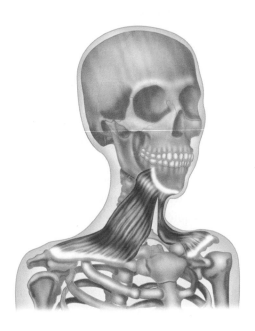

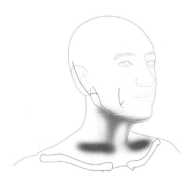

Greek, *platys*, broad, flat.

Origin
Skin and superficial fascia of the neck and upper quarter of the chest, and sometimes out to the shoulder.

Insertion
Subcutaneous fascia of the chin and jaw, including the associated muscles.

Nerve
Facial nerve VII (cervical branch).

Action
Assists in opening the mouth and produces an expression of effort or horror. Pulls the lower lip from the corner of the mouth down and out to the side.

Kinetic Chain Comment
Platysma is a muscle of the integumentary system and is used by horses to shake off irritating insects. Hypertension in this muscle pulls the mouth downward and the thoracic skin forward. It is considered that tissues overlying the thyroid gland might have an influence on glandular function, and so should be examined when glandular dysfunctions are noted. Referral is recommended. This muscle is often punished when exerting fatigue sets in, because of neuromuscular inefficiency or lack of fitness, leading to strain being placed on platysma. A short, tight masseter can inhibit platysma, resulting in teeth grinding, especially during sleep.

Myofascial Trigger Point Comment
A hot prickling pain in the upper chest and under the jawbone can be the result of myofascial trigger points in this integumentary muscle. The fibers of platysma blend into the associated muscles of the face and upper chest wall, such as orbicularis oris (mouth), subclavius, and pectorals. Myofascial trigger points can develop, provoking anterior throat stiffness and increased blinking of the eyelids.

Practitioner Guidelines
Patient positioning
Patient is supine or side lying, with the head rotated to the opposite side.

Needle type
Use 0.25 to 0.30 mm × 30 mm needle.

Needling directions
A very shallow approach is taken, with the therapist holding the targeted tissues between their fingers. Keep in mind that this a muscle of the integumentary system.

Precautions
Use a shallow angle of insertion, ensuring not to place the needle beyond the subcutis.

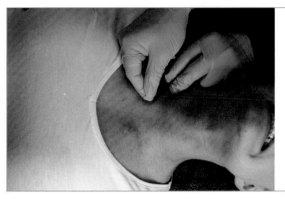 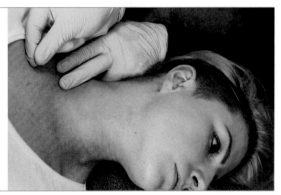

Platysma, supine.

HYOIDS

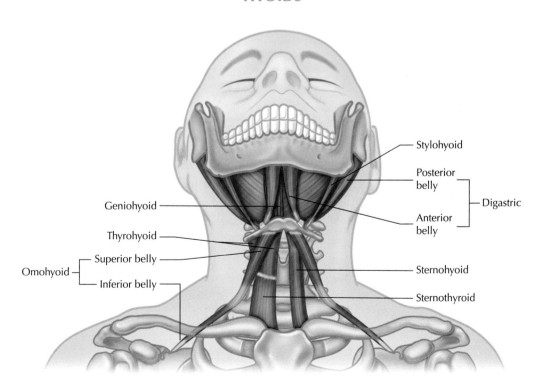

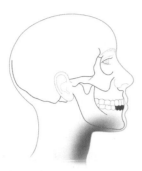

Hyoids referred pain pattern

Greek, *hyoeides*, shaped like the Greek letter upsilon (υ), *omos*, shoulder; *hyoeides*, shaped like the Greek letter upsilon (υ).

Origin

The many muscles of the hyoid group have attachments to the mandible, the temporal bone, the manubrium, the clavicle, the costal cartilage of the first rib, and the thyroid cartilage.

Omohyoid

Posterior belly: Mastoid notch on the mastoid process of the temporal bone.
Anterior belly: Inferior border of the mandible.

Insertion

Hyoid bone.

Nerve

Ansa cervicalis nerve C1–3.

Action

These muscles affect the positioning of the hyoid bone. They particularly offer stiffness to stabilize the hyoid when other muscles are carrying out some function. Omohyoid depresses the hyoid bone.

Kinetic Chain Comment

Mylohyoid, sternohyoid, omohyoid, geniohyoid, sternothyrohyoid, thyrohyoid, stylohyoid, and digastric (indirect attachment)

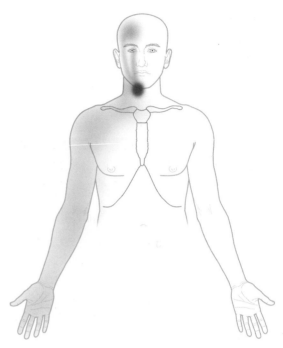

Right omohyoid referral pattern

all contract to hold the hyoid in place when performing supine sit-ups. They can only do this effectively if the tongue, which also attaches to the hyoid, is held in its physiological resting position in the roof of the mouth.

Omohyoid can literally pick up the lungs, as its superior transverse ligament has a fascial connection to the apex of that organ. The hyoids are important muscles in forced inspiration. If they cannot provide the necessary forces, it is easy to assume an individual would have difficulty improving their aerobic fitness or have difficulty breathing when under stress or increased intensity because of physical activity.

Omohyoid eccentrically decelerates the tilting of the head to the contralateral side and the depression of the scapula.

Myofascial Trigger Point Comment

Myofascial trigger points can form in the hyoids, referring pain into the lower front teeth and throughout the cervical spine, mostly as anterior neck pain. I suggest that myofascial trigger points can develop in these muscles because of inhibited transversus abdominis and obliquus internus abdominis, coupled with spastic sternocleidomastoid and suboccipital muscles, caused by faulty training.

Relating to omohyoid, patients often complain of sore throats and difficulty swallowing. My experience has been that this muscle can send pain into the shoulder and up into the head on the same side. Tenderness on the hyoid bone itself is noted. Pain in the shoulder, neck, arm, and hand, as well as in the scapular, supraclavicular, mandibular, and temporal regions, may be caused by the omohyoid. The pain may be primary, caused by vomiting or by some other intense use of the muscle.

Caution: Myofascial trigger points may be secondary, occurring due to rheumatoid myositis, ankylosing spondylitis, non-ankylosing rheumatoid spondylitis, gouty myositis, or other disorders, which should be ruled out in the first instance.

Practitioner Guidelines

Patient positioning
Patient is supine or side lying, with the head rotated to the opposite side.

Needle type
Use 0.14 to 0.16 mm × 15 mm needle.

Needling directions
A very shallow approach is taken, with the therapist palpating the targeted tissues beneath their fingers. A slight change of angle is required to direct the needle toward a specific infra- or supra-hyoid muscle. The image used shows one possible approach. Care must be taken to avoid placing the needle deep in the anterior cervical region.

Precautions
Use a shallow angle of insertion, ensuring not to place the needle overly deep.

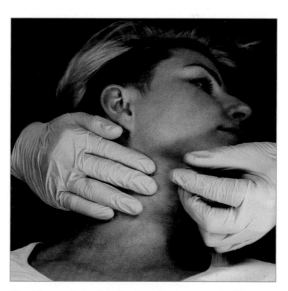

Hyoids, supine with the head rotated to facilitate access to these muscles.

DIGASTRICUS

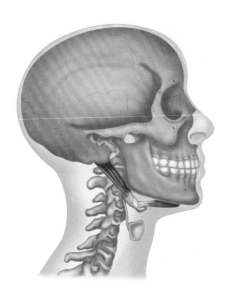

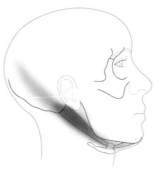

Left posterior digastric TrP referral pattern

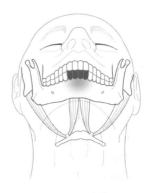

Anterior digastric TrP referral pattern

Latin, *digastricus*, having two (muscle) bellies.

Along with stylohyoid, mylohyoid, and geniohyoid, a suprahyoid muscle (therefore lying above the hyoid bone).

Origin
Anterior belly: Digastric fossa on the inner side of the lower border of the mandible, close to the symphysis.

Posterior belly: Mastoid notch of temporal bone.

Insertion
Body of the hyoid bone, by means of a fascial sling over its intermediate tendon.

Nerve
Anterior belly: Mylohyoid nerve, from trigeminal V nerve (mandibular division).

Posterior belly: Facial (VII) nerve.

Action
Raises the hyoid bone. Depresses and retracts the mandible.

Kinetic Chain Comment
Digastricus must be allowed to create appropriate tension during movements such as crunches or sit-ups. When the tongue is not placed in its physiological resting position, digastricus cannot create this tension, causing sternocleidomastoid to stiffen and shorten—resulting in a forward-head posture—leading to myofascial trigger points down the kinetic chain.

Myofascial Trigger Point Comment
Pain is experienced in the front teeth and anterior jawbone, and into the upper part of sternocleidomastoid (occasionally onto the base of the occiput) and into the throat under the chin. Digastric myofascial trigger points have been reported to be responsible for satellite myofascial trigger points in occipitofrontalis and for referring pain into the ear.

Practitioner Guidelines

Patient positioning
Patient is supine or side lying, with the head rotated to the opposite side.

Needle type
Use 0.25 to 0.30 mm × 30 mm needle.

Needling directions
A very shallow approach is taken, with the therapist holding the targeted tissues between their fingers. Direct the needle toward the mastoid process, or in the opposite direction toward the mental spines. Other associated muscle fibers may be needled due to their proximity, e.g., mylohyoid.

Precautions
Use a shallow angle of insertion.

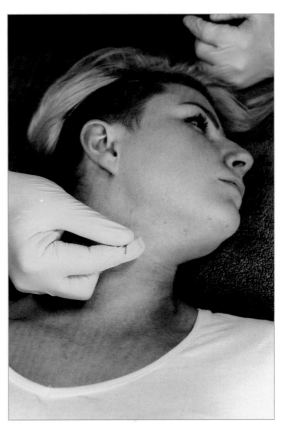

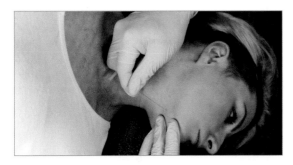

Digastricus (anterior), supine.

Digastricus (posterior), supine.

LONGUS COLLI

Latin, *longus*, long; *colli*, of the neck.

Origin
Longus colli has three specific parts—superior oblique, inferior oblique, vertical—lying on the anterior lateral aspect of both the upper cervical and thoracic vertebrae. The origin ranges from the transverse processes of C3–5 with attachments to the anterior aspects of C1–2 and including the anterior surface of the T1–3.

Insertion
Anterior tubercle of the atlas, and anterior tubercles of the transverse processes C5, C6.

Nerve
Ventral rami of cervical nerves C2–7.

Action
Bilaterally flexes the cervical spine, while unilateral contraction assists in rotation to the opposite side and lateral neck flexion.

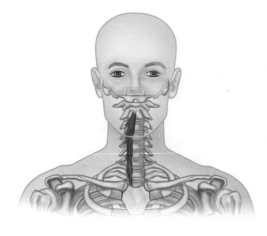

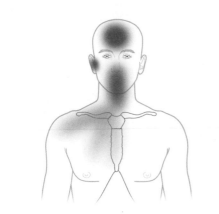

Kinetic Chain Comment

Longus colli becomes short and tight because of inappropriate neck movements resulting in short scalenes as well as a short, tight psoas, which in turn affects the action of the diaphragm, thereby leading to myofascial trigger point formations that cause neck, upper back, and lower back pain. Longus colli bilaterally decelerates extension of the neck, and unilaterally decelerates ipsilateral rotation and lateral neck extension.

Myofascial Trigger Point Comment

Common symptoms are problems with swallowing, pain in the anterior neck, mouth, ear, and head, and a feeling of a lump in the throat. Patients may complain of a sore throat. I have experienced myofascial trigger points that refer pain across the upper chest on the affected side to the ipsilateral deltoid and produce a feeling of tightness across the chest. Patients also report pain across the anterior clavicle and into the tongue.

A short spastic psoas can have a significant effect on the development of myofascial trigger points in longus colli and associated muscles of the neck. Local pain is reported as a deep, thin, and acute sensation at the vertebral level, rising to the eye on the ipsilateral side. Longus colli can be the true source of sternocleidomastoid pain and is worth considering for treatment in sternocleidomastoid pain issues.

Practitioner Guidelines
Patient positioning
Patient is supine or side lying, with the head rotated to the opposite side.

Needle type
Use 0.14 to 0.16 mm × 15 mm needle.

Needling directions
A very shallow approach is taken, with the therapist holding the targeted tissues beneath their fingers.

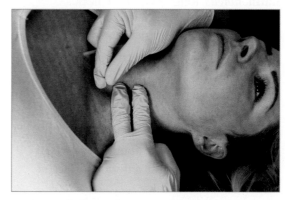

Supine with the trachea moved laterally.

Precautions
This muscle requires advanced palpation skills and excellent anatomical knowledge. Structures in this area are many, including the common carotid artery, internal jugular vein, vagus nerve (CN X), and the deep cervical lymph nodes. The therapist must move the trachea and associated structures to the opposite side to allow space for needle insertion. Work slowly and with caution, guiding the needle in an inferior to superior direction, and in a medial to lateral direction.

LONGUS CAPITIS

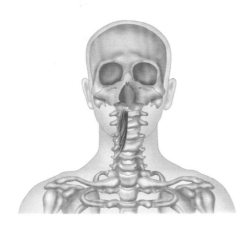

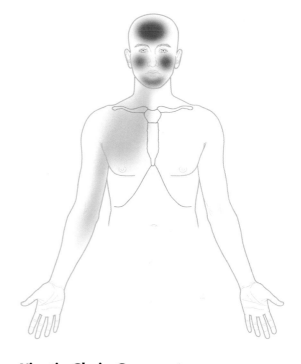

Latin, *longus*, long; *capitis*, of the head.

Origin
Anterior tubercles of the transverse processes of C3–6.

Insertion
Inferior surface of the basilar portion of the occiput.

Nerve
Ventral rami of cervical nerves C1–4.

Action
Flexes the neck and superior portion of the cervical spine.

Kinetic Chain Comment
Longus capitis decelerates neck extension. It may be worth treating short psoas muscles as part of the treatment of longus capitis since myofascial trigger points can be formed as a response to spasm in the lower chain muscles.

Myofascial Trigger Point Comment
Longus capitis can contribute to general pain in the head, face, teeth, and jaw while referring

pain down the arm and chest wall. Patients experience pain in the front of the throat and complain of difficulty swallowing. A feeling of a lump in the throat and sinus-type pain is reported.

Practitioner Guidelines

Patient positioning
Patient is supine or side lying, with the head rotated to the opposite side.

Needle type
Use 0.25 to 0.30 mm × 30 mm needle.

Needling directions
Therapist moves the trachea laterally and engages the muscle with their fingertips, locating the taut band and nodules.

Precautions
Use a lateral to medial direction for insertion.

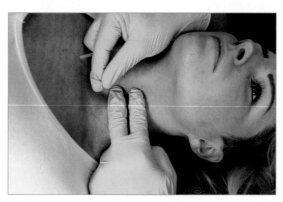

Longus colli and capitis, supine.

RECTUS CAPITIS (ANTERIOR, LATERALIS)

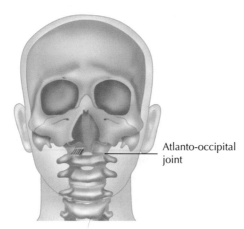

Rectus capitis anterior

Atlanto-occipital joint

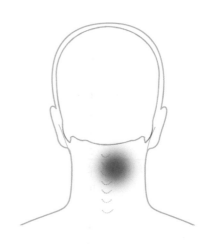

Latin, *rectus*, straight; *capitis*, of the head; *anterior*, at the front; *lateral*, relating to the side.

Origin
Anterior: Anterior surface of the lateral mass of the atlas.
Lateralis: Transverse process of the atlas.

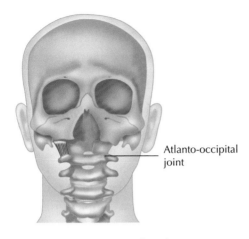

Rectus capitis lateralis

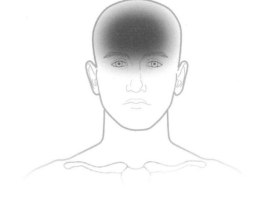

Atlanto-occipital joint

Insertion

Anterior: Basilar portion.
Lateralis: Jugular process.

Nerve

Loop between the ventral rami of cervical nerves C1, C2.

Action

Anterior: Flexes the head.
Lateralis: Lateral flexion to the same side.

Kinetic Chain Comment

Rectus capitis decelerates the head during extension and contralateral flexion. Spasm or shortness in this muscle can set up the foundation for retarded proprioceptive facilitation and a tendency to collide with objects, get timing wrong, and reduce accuracy. Attention should be paid to the sternocleidomastoid and head position, in conjunction with a focus on the posterior myofascial chain. Remember, from a kinetic chain viewpoint, the true source of rectus capitis dysfunction could be as far away as the plantar fascia.

Myofascial Trigger Point Comment

Myofascial trigger points in this muscle can feel like severe migraine-type pain everywhere inside the head. Patients may say they cannot pinpoint the pain but feel it widespread throughout the cranium. As in other posterior neck muscles, these myofascial trigger points can contribute to painful tension-like or cervicogenic headaches; the eyes become sensitive to bright light, and patients experience difficulty concentrating. Changes in sensations can include numbness, tingling, and burning in the scalp. Myofascial trigger points can reduce or retard blood flow and impede nerve tissue.

Practitioner Guidelines

It is not recommended to dry needle this muscle, because of the proximity of the vertebral artery. However, although the muscles cannot be dry needled, the therapist can use their fingers or thumb to relieve any trigger point formation.

SCALENES

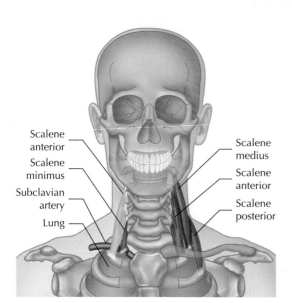

Greek, *skalenos*, uneven.

Origin
Transverse processes of all cervical vertebrae.

Insertion
First rib and/or suprapleural membrane. Posterior portion may attach to the first two ribs.

Nerve
Ventral rami of cervical nerves C3–8.

Action
Elevates the ribs for respiration if the ribs are fixed. Rotates to the side opposite to the muscle contracting. Laterally flexes to the contracted side. Bilaterally flexes the neck.

Kinetic Chain Comment
Myofascial trigger points causing short psoas muscles can lead to adaptations in scalenes, resulting in a short, contracted state, thereby pulling up the ribcage and affecting respiratory efficiency.

Myofascial Trigger Point Comment
Pain and numbness can be experienced in the anterior chest, the upper back, and the lateroanterior shoulder down the arm, radiating into the thumb and second digit. These are a complex group of muscles with varying muscle fiber lengths, and therefore demonstrate the potential for many myofascial trigger points. Excellent palpatory skills will be required to successfully locate such myofascial trigger points.

Practitioner Guidelines
Patient positioning
Patient is supine or side lying, with the head rotated to the opposite side.

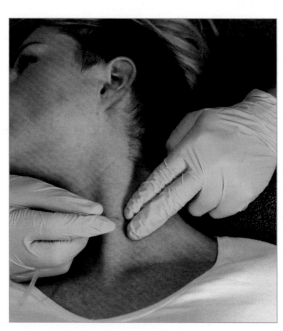

Supine with the head rotated.

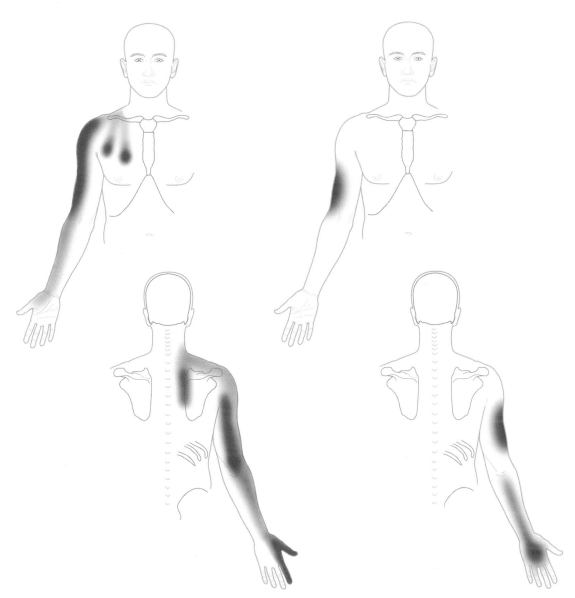

Combined referral pattern for scalenes medius, anterior, and posterior, which, together, are called the scalene major

Combined referral pattern for scalene minimus

Needle type
Use 0.25 to 0.30 mm × 30 mm needle.

Needling directions
Direct the needle posterior to the sternocleidomastoid, moving in an anterior to posterior direction.

Precautions
Care must be taken to avoid neurovascular tissues (e.g., the carotid artery) and to insert the needle well above the apex of the lung (two finger widths above the clavicle are recommended).

STERNOCLEIDOMASTOID

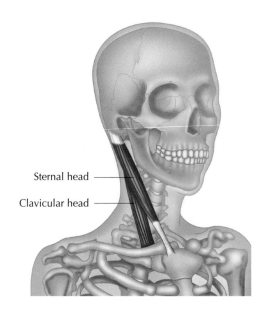

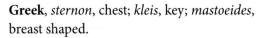

Sternal head

Clavicular head

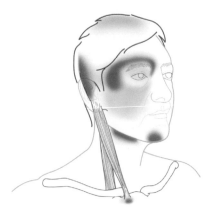

Sternal division

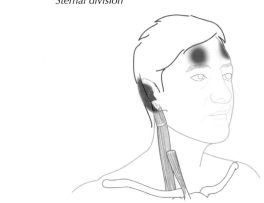

Clavicular division

Greek, *sternon*, chest; *kleis*, key; *mastoeides*, breast shaped.

Origin
Manubrium of the sternum and medial portion of the clavicle (two heads).

Insertion
Mastoid process of the temporal bone.

Nerve
Accessory XI nerve, with sensory supply for proprioception from cervical nerves C2, C3.

Action
Rotates head to the side opposite that contracting and laterally flexes to the contracted side. Bilaterally flexes the cervical spine (neck).

Kinetic Chain Comment
Generally, sternocleidomastoid is the muscle that most people feel hurting or tense when performing sit-ups. When short, it changes the position of the head on the neck, resulting in a forward-head posture; this sets up the foundation for kinetic chain pain and postural changes, leading to compensation, change of gait, and decompensation. Rounded shoulders often have their roots in a short sternocleidomastoid.

Myofascial Trigger Point Comment
Sternocleidomastoid symptoms include problems with balance, visual difficulties, and headache. Because of their anatomical position, myofascial trigger points in this muscle can be mistaken for swollen glands.

Referred pain can be felt as a headache across the front of the brow, deep eye pain (involving decreased or blurred vision), pain on swallowing, and pain behind the ear (including a degree of deafness) and in the top (crown) of the head.

I have had patients with sternocleidomastoid myofascial trigger points who experienced pain similar to trigeminal neuralgia; such pain can be diagnosed as sinusitis. Rare pain referral can also include toothache in the back molars, and pain on the opposite side of the forehead. Pain in the manubrium of the sternum has also been reported. Pain is referred to the temples, tongue, and throat, and to the side of the neck in some patients.

Practitioner Guidelines
Patient positioning
Patient is supine.

Needle type
Use 0.25 to 0.30 mm × 30 mm needle.

Needling directions
I recommend a pincer grip of this muscle. Remember, the needle can pass through to the outside, which poses the risk to the therapist of needle stick. Be mindful at all times of finger and thumb placement.

Precautions
Locate and avoid the carotid artery, which is located medially to this muscle, between the trachea and medial border of the sternocleidomastoid. Avoiding pressing too hard on the carotid artery, as this closes it, and the therapist will then not be able to locate the pulse. Land softly on the skin and listen with the flat pads of your first and second digits. Using a pincer grip as shown allows the therapist to dissociate this muscle from the associated neurovascular structures. Use a tangential angle of insertion in a medial to lateral direction and an anterior to posterior direction.

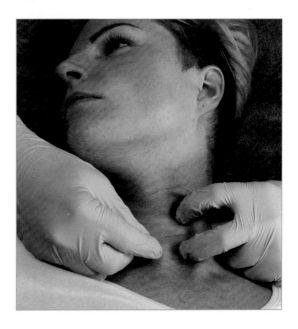

SUBOCCIPITAL GROUP

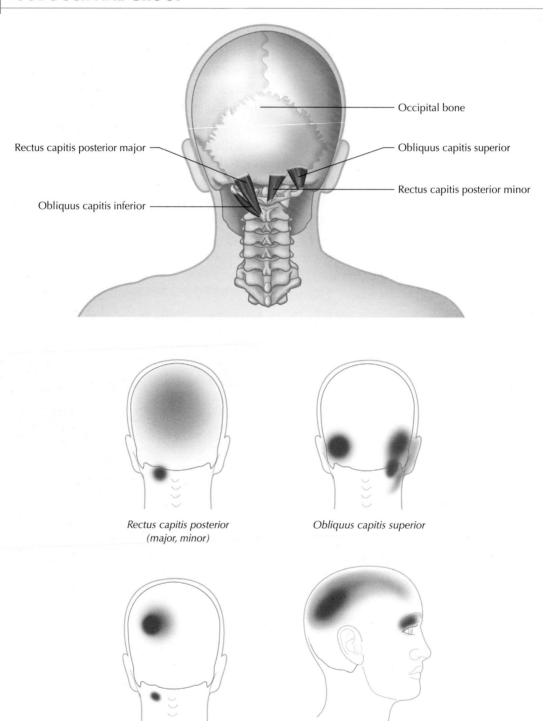

Occipital bone

Rectus capitis posterior major

Obliquus capitis superior

Obliquus capitis inferior

Rectus capitis posterior minor

Rectus capitis posterior
(major, minor)

Obliquus capitis superior

Obliquus capitis inferior

RECTUS CAPITIS POSTERIOR (MAJOR, MINOR)

Latin, *rectus*, straight; *capitis*, of the head; *posterior*, at the back; *major*, larger; *minor*, smaller.

Origin
Posterior process of the atlas (C1).

Insertion
Medial half of the inferior nuchal line.

Nerve
Suboccipital nerve (dorsal ramus of first cervical nerve C1).

Action
Extend and rotate the atlanto-occipital joint.

Kinetic Chain Comment
These muscles form part of the suboccipital group and are vital for reporting the position of the body in time and space. They are rich in muscle spindles, and their role is as much about sending information to the brain regarding head position, as it is about creating movement. With fascial attachments to the spinal cord and brain via the dura mater, these muscles are vital to spinal health and the healthy flow of cerebrospinal fluid.

Myofascial Trigger Point Comment
Mimicking migraine pain, these muscles often create what many patients refer to as "brain pain." A pain is felt deep in the head, but the patient cannot put their finger on exactly where the pain is. Migraine pain has often been attributed to these muscles.

Practitioner Guidelines
Patient positioning
Patient is prone. Head rotation is optional.

Needle type
Use 0.25 to 0.30 mm × 30 mm needle.

Needling directions
Extra caution is required when needling the suboccipital muscles: the therapist must ensure that they are always aware of the depth of the needle. Needling in an inferior to superior direction and lateral to medial direction is recommended. Direct the needle toward the opposite eye.

Precautions
Use a tangential angle of insertion, directing the needle toward the eye on the opposite side. Expert knowledge of anatomy is required.

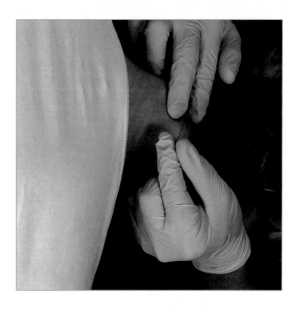

OBLIQUUS CAPITIS INFERIOR

Latin, *obliquus*, diagonal, slanted; *capitis*, of the head; *inferior*, lower.

Origin
Spinous process of the axis (C2).

Insertion
Lateral mass of the atlas (C1).

Nerve
Suboccipital nerve (dorsal ramus of first cervical nerve C1).

Action
Rotates the atlanto-axial joint.

Kinetic Chain Comment
Any small change in head position will ultimately affect the status of this muscle.

Myofascial Trigger Point Comment
Pain shooting from the back of the head into the eye is a regular complaint of headache, particularly migraine, sufferers. As this is the pain referral of the obliquus capitis inferior, it should be included as part of any treatment plan for patients complaining of similar patterns.

Practitioner Guidelines
Patient positioning
Patient is prone.

Needle type
Use 0.25 to 0.30 mm × 30 mm needle.

Needling directions
Extra caution is required when needling the suboccipital muscles: the therapist must ensure that they are always aware of the depth of the needle. Needling in an inferior to superior direction and lateral to medial direction is recommended. Direct the needle toward the opposite eye.

Precautions
Use a tangential angle of insertion, directing the needle toward the eye on the opposite side. Expert knowledge of anatomy is required. While the application of the needle insertion and precautions are like those for the rectus capitis posterior (major, minor), the therapist must possess the necessary palpation skills to locate the various suboccipital muscles—in this case, the ones located more laterally.

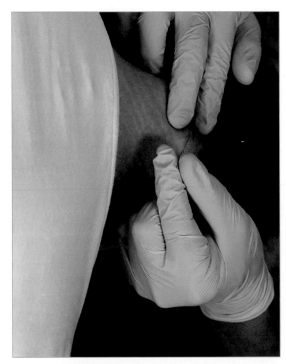

To target obliquus capitis inferior, angle the needle in a more lateral direction.

OBLIQUUS CAPITIS SUPERIOR

Latin, *obliquus*, diagonal, slanting; *capitis*, of the head; *superior*, upper.

Origin
Lateral mass of the transverse process of the atlas (C1).

Insertion
Lateral half of the inferior nuchal line.

Nerve
Suboccipital nerve (dorsal ramus of first cervical nerve C1).

Action
Laterally flexes the atlanto-occipital joint.

Kinetic Chain Comment
Decelerates flexion and contralateral extension of the head at the neck. Obliquus capitis superior and inferior are enriched with muscle spindles, and their positioning is very important to achieving efficient posture.

Myofascial Trigger Point Comment
Obliquus capitis superior will cause dull, deep pain over the lateral aspects of the occipital bone, with diffuse pain radiating down the sides of the jawbone and into the ears.

Practitioner Guidelines
It is not recommended to dry needle this muscle, because of the proximity of the vertebral artery. However, although the muscles cannot be dry needled, the therapist can use their fingers or thumb to relieve any trigger point formation.

Muscles of the Trunk and Spine

ERECTOR SPINAE (SACROSPINALIS)

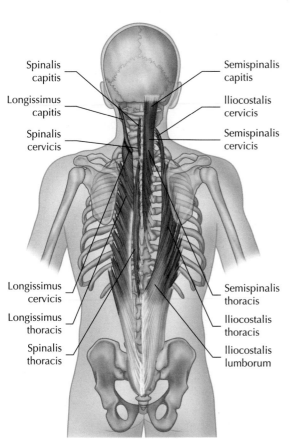

Spinalis capitis

Longissimus capitis

Spinalis cervicis

Semispinalis capitis

Iliocostalis cervicis

Semispinalis cervicis

Longissimus cervicis

Longissimus thoracis

Spinalis thoracis

Semispinalis thoracis

Iliocostalis thoracis

Iliocostalis lumborum

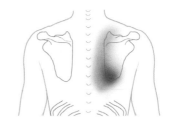

Upper iliocostalis posterior referral pattern

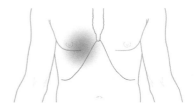

Upper iliocostalis anterior referral pattern

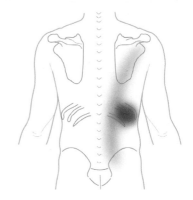

Posterior iliocostalis thoracis referral pattern

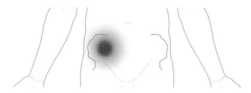

Anterior iliocostalis thoracis referral pattern

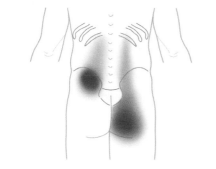

Lower thoracic longissimus thoracis referral pattern

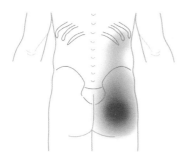

Iliocostalis lumborum referral pattern

Latin, *erigere*, to erect; *spinae*, of the spine; *sacrum*, sacred; *spinalis*, relating to the spine.

Origin
Each of the many erector spinae muscles conjoin with the thoracolumbar fascia that attaches at several different angles to the crest of the ilium and sacrum, and to the spinous processes of T11–12 and L1–5.

Insertion
Many different attachments to the posterior costal bones, the spinous and transverse processes of the thoracic and cervical vertebrae, and the mastoid process of the temporal bone.

Nerve
Dorsal rami of cervical, thoracic, and lumbar spinal nerves.

Action
Extends the vertebral column while the deep rotators and multifidi erectors rotate the spinal column to the opposite side. The semispinalis extends the vertebral column and the head.

Kinetic Chain Comment
This group includes the iliocostalis, longissimus, spinalis, and multifidi. Eccentrically, these muscles decelerate forward flexion, lateral flexion, and rotation. These muscles are the main stabilizers of the lumbar spine in normal gait.

Myofascial Trigger Point Comment
Refer pain from the lumbar erectors into the gluteal and sacral areas. As a loose rule, pain generally refers up and out, with myofascial trigger points in the suboccipitals, causing severe headaches. Mid-thoracic myofascial trigger points can refer pain into the anterior chest wall and abdomen. Pain experienced as rib pain can often be related to myofascial trigger points. Myofascial trigger points in the cervical spine are often caused by repeated supine sit-ups or crunches performed on the floor, without first stabilizing the hyoid by means of correct tongue position. These in turn can perpetuate myofascial trigger points in the psoas, scalenes, and sternocleidomastoid, and down the chain into the plantars.

Practitioner Guidelines

Patient positioning
Patient is prone.

Needle type
Use 0.25 to 0.30 mm × 30 mm needle.

Needling directions
Care is required to work within the lamina groove. Stay within a finger width lateral to the spinous process in the safe needling zone, ensuring that there is no rotation of the vertebral body when needling the erector spinae muscles. The various laterally placed erector spinae muscles, including longissimus and iliocostalis, require attention to identify the ribs. The therapist should needle over the ribs to avoid penetrating the lung with the needle.

Precautions
Locate the lamina groove.

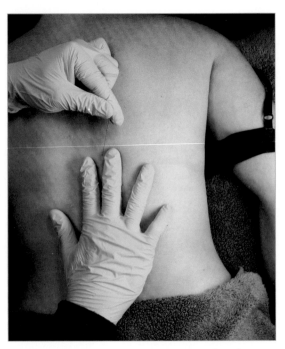

Needle in the lamina groove, ensuring that there is no rotation of the vertebrae.

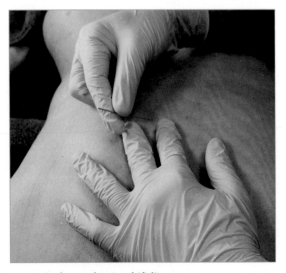

Paraspinal muscles (multifidi), prone.

SPLENIUS CAPITIS

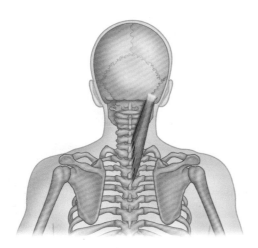

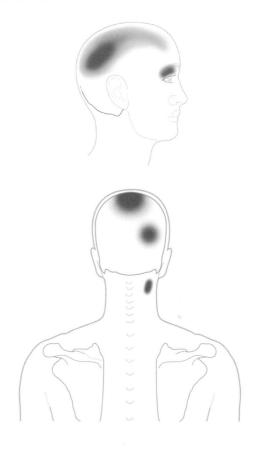

Greek, *splenion*, bandage. **Latin**, *capitis*, of the head.

Origin
Inferior aspect of the ligamentum nuchae, and spinous processes of C7 and T1–4.

Insertion
Mastoid process (posterior portion).

Nerve
Dorsal rami of middle and lower cervical nerves.

Action
Bilaterally extends the head and neck. Ipsilaterally flexes and rotates the neck.

Kinetic Chain Comment
Poor computer positioning or poor posture when reading can lead to stress of the splenius capitis. Eyes positioned below the level of a computer screen require the operator to look up, activating these muscles and over time creating a hyperextended cervical spine. This requires the pelvis to tilt anteriorly to flex the head so that the eyes can once again be level.

Myofascial Trigger Point Comment
All the muscles of the posterior cervical spine should be investigated when patients complain of tension-type headaches. Splenius capitis is yet another contributor of referred pain into the skull. Any head movement will involve this muscle in any one of a number of ways; it is therefore an important muscle in ensuring appropriate head positioning. Pain spreads up to the crown of the head and into the back of the ipsilateral eye (similarly to the sternocleidomastoid). Blurred vision and a headache with explosive pressure in the eye are often reported. Once serious eye pathologies have been ruled out, myofascial trigger points are the most likely cause of complaint.

Practitioner Guidelines

Patient positioning
Patient is side lying.

Needle type
Use 0.25 to 0.30 mm × 30 mm needle.

Needling directions
Direct the needle toward the mastoid process, staying posterior to the transverse process.

Precautions
Keep the needle at a shallow angle.

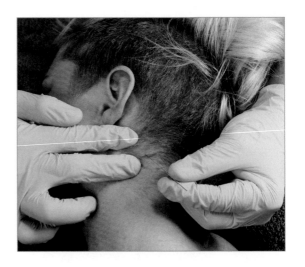

SPLENIUS CERVICIS

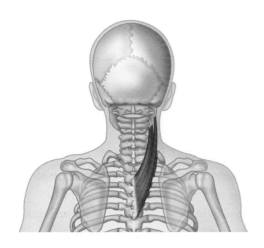

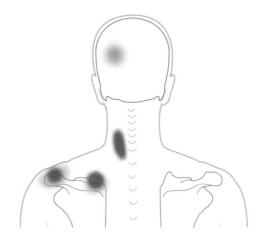

Greek, *splenion*, bandage. **Latin**, *cervicis*, of the neck.

Origin
Ligamentum nuchae, and spinous process of C7.

Insertion
Spinous process of C2 (axis).

Nerve
Dorsal rami of spinal nerves.

Action
Extends the vertebral column. Keeps the spine upright, giving lift when standing.

Kinetic Chain Comment
The cervical muscles—including splenius cervicis—are as important to full-body movement as they are to core musculature.

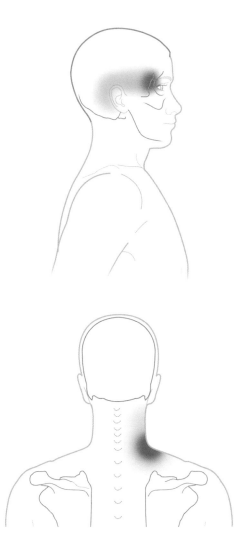

acromion process. Myofascial trigger points in this muscle contribute to tension-type headaches, with pain felt over the temporal and occipital bones.

Practitioner Guidelines
Patient positioning
Patient is side lying.

Needle type
Use 0.25 to 0.30 mm × 30 mm needle.

Needling directions
Identify the myofascial trigger point and direct the needle, as shown in the image, between the therapist's fingers, only to the depth of the muscle, in a lateral to medial direction.

Precautions
To eliminate risks, needle in an anterior to posterior direction, as shown in the image.

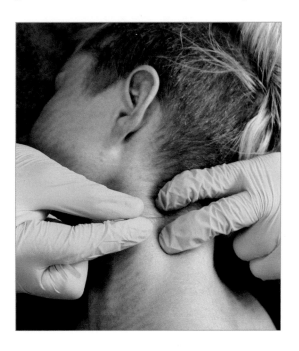

A short splenius cervicis can displace the cervical or thoracic vertebrae, thereby affecting fourth-layer muscles (splenii, semispinalis, multifidus, and rotatores) and the positioning of the thoracic ribs. Such changes result in postural adaptations up and down the kinetic chain.

Myofascial Trigger Point Comment
Pain is referred down onto the superior angle of the scapula and anteriorly out to the

LONGISSIMUS CAPITIS

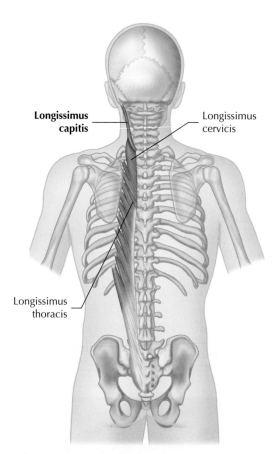

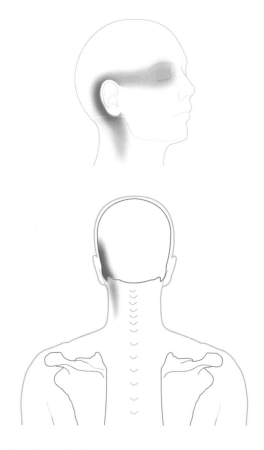

Latin, *longissimus*, longest; *capitis*, of the head.

Origin
Upper five transverse processes of the thoracic vertebrae and articular processes of C5–7.

Insertion
Posterior margin of the mastoid process.

Nerve
Dorsal rami of middle and lower cervical nerves.

Action
This deep neck muscle extends the head and rotates the face toward the ipsilateral side.

Kinetic Chain Comment
Because of its proximity to important neurovascular structures, longissimus capitis is an ideal muscle to use as an example of the need for differential diagnosis and of the necessity to work within a multidisciplinary context, referring when in any doubt.

Pain, referred or otherwise, in this area could be a result of the following: degenerative disc disease (segmental, subluxation, somatic dysfunction), C2/3 radiculopathy (bulging, prolapsed, herniated disc), fibromyalgia, osteoporosis, osteoarthritis, rheumatoid arthritis, intervertebral or vertebral stenosis, vertebral vascular disorder, cerebral aneurysm, cerebral neoplasm (brain cancer), military neck (absence of normal cervical spine lordosis), cervical spine hyperlordosis, thoracic spine hyperkyphosis, scoliosis, tension/cluster headaches, suboccipital articular dysfunction, mastoiditis, cervical arthritis, cervical syndrome, subacute meningitis, polymyalgia rheumatica, polymyositis, systemic lupus erythematosus, acceleration/deceleration injury (whiplash), eye strain, ocular disease, sinusitis, tetanus, systemic infections or inflammation, nutritional inadequacy, metabolic imbalance, or toxicity or side effects of medications.

Appropriate screening will provide you with the necessary information to decide when to refer. Remember, if in doubt, refer.

Myofascial Trigger Point Comment
Pain referred from this muscle travels to the posterior aspect of the ear. The pain can also extend somewhat across the neck and behind the eyes. Myofascial trigger points in this muscle contribute to headache pain, with tenderness reported at the occipital bone and upper neck, sometimes accompanied by numbness and tingling in the scalp.

Practitioner Guidelines
Patient positioning
Patient is prone.

Needle type
Use 0.25 to 0.30 mm × 30 mm needle.

Needling directions
Needle in a superior to inferior direction.

Precautions
Ensure that you work above the first rib (to avoid any possibility of a pneumothorax) staying within the borders of C6 to C2 as far out as the transverse processes (articulating pillars) or no more than one finger's width out and direct the needle at a shallow angle toward the lamina working lateral to medial, superior to inferior.

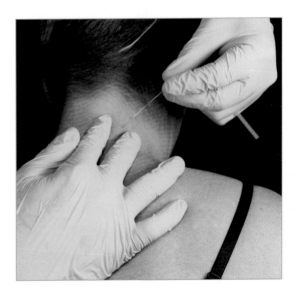

MULTIFIDUS

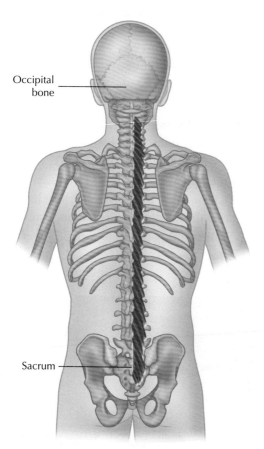

Occipital bone

Sacrum

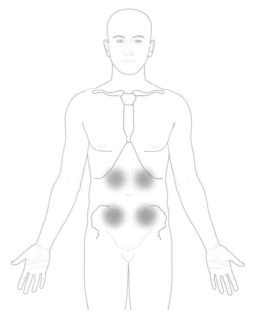

Anterior multifidi referral patterns

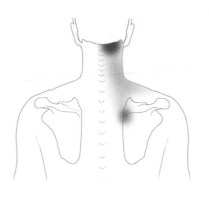

Cervical multifidi

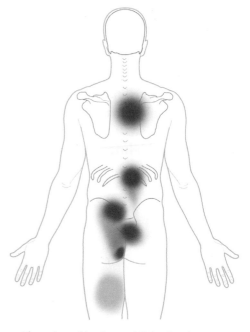

Thoracic and lumbar multifidi referral patterns

Latin, *multi*, many, much; *findere*, to split.

Origin
Posterior aspect of the iliac crest and sacrum, sacroiliac ligament, mammillary process of the lumbar vertebrae, and transverse processes of the thoracic vertebrae, including articular processes of C4–7.

Insertion
Spinous processes of superior vertebrae.

Nerve
Dorsal rami of spinal nerves.

Action
Extends, laterally flexes, and rotates the vertebral column, in addition to extending and laterally rotating the pelvis. A core fourth-layer muscle.

Kinetic Chain Comment
A major contributor to neuromuscular efficiency of the "core." The deep multifidus has a role in controlling intersegmental motion.

Note: Spinal integrity relies on the combined ability of all muscles; however, special consideration should be given to the transversus abdominis muscle in maintaining pelvic stability, and to the action of multifidus and rotatores in stabilizing the spinal structure.

Myofascial Trigger Point Comment
Pain is reported at the spinous processes of L1–5 and anterior to the abdomen. S1 projects pain down to the coccyx; this referral radiates laterally from the level of T4–5 to the inferior angle of the scapula. Myofascial trigger points located in the cervical region of the multifidus refer pain from the suboccipital region, down the posterior neck to the approximate segmental level of T3 and laterally to the rhomboids. There is also a lateral distribution at the base of the neck and upper back region.

Practitioner Guidelines
Patient positioning
Patient is prone.

Needle type
Use 0.25 to 0.30 mm × 30 mm needle.

Needling directions
Needle in an inferior direction, within a finger width of the spinous process (i.e., lamina groove).

Precautions
Needle slowly, always looking for patient feedback.

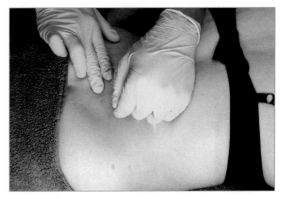

Working slowly is essential: if the needle approaches any nerve structure, the patient will be able to inform the therapist whenever the therapist is working slowly. Speed is the enemy. The needle is directed medially and inferiorly (caudally).

ROTATORES

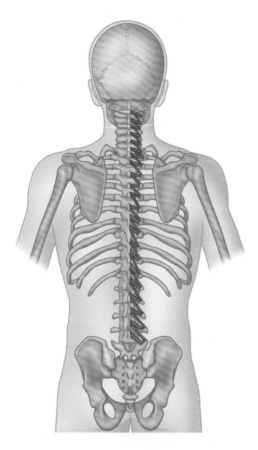

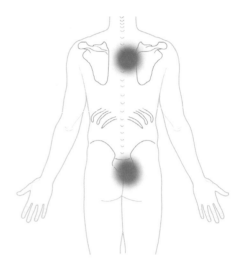

Latin, *rota*, wheel.

Origin
(Eleven pairs from the sacrum to C2).
Transverse process (inferior).

Insertion
Spinous process (superior).

Nerve
Posterior rami of the thoracic nerves.

Action
Extend and rotate the vertebrae.

Kinetic Chain Comment
A major muscle in neuromuscular efficiency
of the "core."

Note: Spinal integrity relies on the combined
ability of all muscles; however, special
consideration should be given to the
transversus abdominis muscle in maintaining
pelvic stability, and to the action of multifidus
and rotatores in stabilizing the spinal
structure.

Myofascial Trigger Point Comment
In my years of human cadaver studies, I have
seen no need to separate the rotatores from the
multifidi when dealing with myofascial trigger
points. These muscles are basal skull pain
generators as well as neck and scapular pain
generators. Dry needling is, in my opinion,
the most effective method for accessing and
treating these muscles.

Practitioner Guidelines
Patient positioning
Patient is prone.

Needle type
Use 0.25 to 0.30 mm × 30 mm needle.

Needling directions
Needle in an inferior direction, within a finger width of the spinous process (i.e., lamina groove).

Precautions
Direct the needle in a lateral to medial direction and be aware of needle depth.

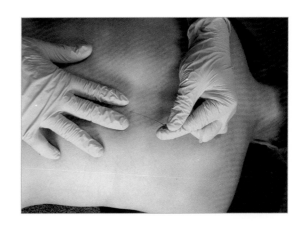

INTERCOSTALS

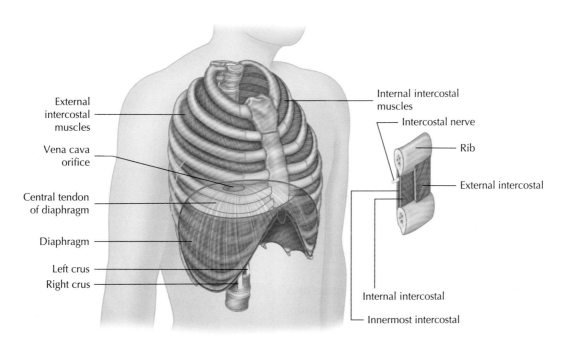

Latin, *inter*, between; *costa*, rib; *externi*, external; *interni*, internal.

Origin
Inferior border of the ribs, as far back as the posterior angles.

Insertion
Superior border of the ribs below, passing obliquely downward and backward.

Nerve
Muscular collateral branches of intercostal nerves.

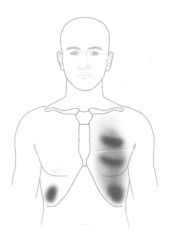

Action

Fix the intercostal spaces during respiration. Aid forced inspiration by elevating the ribs.

Kinetic Chain Comment

These are the principal muscles of respiration. Problems with these muscles can literally change the internal pH of the body. The intercostals draw the central tendon downward during resting respiration. These muscles will also affect frontal plane movement along the lateral line.

Myofascial Trigger Point Comment

Difficulty breathing is reported, with sharp pain felt, particularly on exhaling. Exercise- or activity-induced breathing difficulties can lead to myofascial trigger points being mistaken for exercise-induced asthma.

Practitioner Guidelines

Patient positioning

Patient is prone or side lying.

Needle type

Use 0.25 to 0.30 mm × 30 mm needle.

Needling directions

Needling the intercostal muscles requires expert skills, anatomical knowledge, and competence in handling the needle. The depth of needle insertion is paramount to avoid needling the lung, with a resulting pneumothorax. A shallow angle is recommended after needle insertion. Needle in a medial to lateral direction.

Precautions

Ensure that you avoid a pneumothorax by continually checking your anatomical landmarks and the location of the needle.

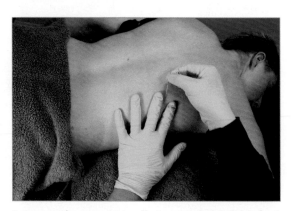

Intercostals, prone. Needle in a medial to lateral direction.

DIAPHRAGM

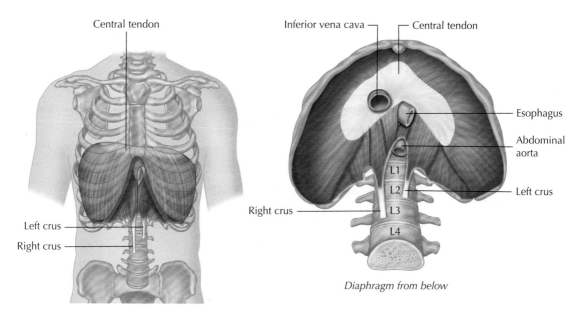

Central tendon

Inferior vena cava — Central tendon

Esophagus

Abdominal aorta

L1

L2 — Left crus

L3

L4

Right crus

Left crus

Right crus

Diaphragm from below

Greek, *dia*, across; *phragma*, partition, wall.

Origin
Sternal portion: Two slips from the posterior aspect of the xiphoid process.
Costal portion: Medial and lateral arcuate ligaments, inner aspect of the lower six ribs.
Lumbar portion: Crura from the bodies of L1–2 (left), L1–3 (right).

Insertion
Central tendon.

Nerve
Phrenic nerve (ventral rami) C3–5.

Action
Inspiration and assists in raising intra-abdominal pressure.

Kinetic Chain Comment
This dome-shaped musculofibrous muscle is penetrated by the aorta, the vena cava, and the esophagus. Fascial investments with the quadratus lumborum and psoas muscles highlight the importance of this structure, linking as it does the lower and upper quarters. The psoas and quadratus lumborum should be treated along with the diaphragm when dealing with respiratory dysfunction.

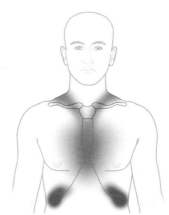

Myofascial Trigger Point Comment
Patients complain of chest pain, dyspnea, and not being able to take a full functional

breath. A stitch in the side is common. Sudden increases in exercise intensity or physical activities can activate, or be the cause of, myofascial trigger point formation in the diaphragm.

Practitioner Guidelines
It is not recommended to dry needle this muscle, because of the proximity of the lungs. However, although this muscle cannot be dry needled, the therapist can use their fingers or thumb to relieve any trigger point formation.

INTERNAL OBLIQUE

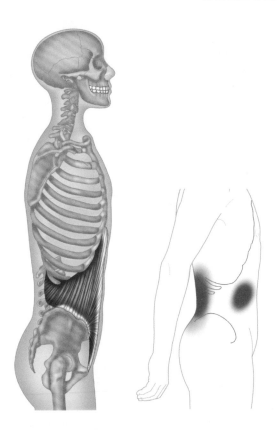

Latin, *obliquus*, diagonal, slanted; *internus*, internal; *abdominis*, of the belly/stomach.

Origin
Lumbar fascia. Anterior two-thirds of the iliac crest, and lateral two-thirds of the inguinal ligament.

Insertion
Costal margin, aponeurosis of the rectus sheath (anterior and posterior), and conjoint tendon to the pubic crest and pectineal line.

Nerve
Ventral rami of thoracic nerves T7–12, ilioinguinal and iliohypogastric nerves.

Action
Supports the abdominal wall, assists forced respiration, and aids in raising intra-abdominal pressure. Along with the muscles of the other side, obliquus internus abdominis abducts and rotates the trunk. The conjoint tendon supports the posterior wall of the inguinal canal.

Kinetic Chain Comment
The most common mistake in exercise programs is the attempt to isolate the internal obliques in relation to the other abdominal muscles, in the exclusion of efforts to train this muscle in the functional manner in which it operates. The internal obliques typically become inhibited when stressed, leading to muscular compensations and changes in pelvic positioning.

Myofascial Trigger Point Comment

Any abdominal pain should be treated with caution. Any suspicion concerning the type of pain or symptoms should be the cue for referral to a doctor. Internal oblique myofascial trigger points refer pain in many directions in the abdomen, including the lower back. Pain across the midline is possible. Patients can complain of burning, bloatedness, and stomach swelling.

Practitioner Guidelines

Patient positioning
Patient is supine.

Needle type
Use 0.25 to 0.30 mm × 30 mm needle.

Needling directions
A tangential approach is required for treating these myofascial trigger points, moving the needle in a medial to lateral direction and an inferior to superior direction.

Precautions
Take a tangential approach to needle insertion and avoid going deeper than the muscle depths. The peritoneal cavity lies deep to the abdominal musculature, and care is required to ensure correct needle depth.

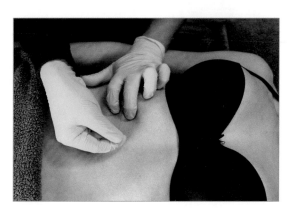

EXTERNAL OBLIQUE

Latin, *obliquus*, diagonal, slanted; *externus*, external; *abdominis*, of the belly/stomach.

Origin
Anterior angles of the lower eight ribs.

Insertion
Outer anterior half of the iliac crest, inguinal ligament, pubic tubercle and crest, and aponeurosis of the anterior rectus sheath.

Nerve
Ventral rami of thoracic nerves T5–12.

Action
Supports the abdominal wall, assists forced expiration, and aids in raising intra-abdominal pressure. Along with the muscles of the opposite side, the obliquus externus abdominis abducts and rotates the trunk.

Kinetic Chain Comment
When considering physical activities to improve the function of the external obliques, one should try to include both open- and closed-kinetic-chain movements.

Myofascial Trigger Point Comment
Pain can refer down into the groin and sometimes to the testicles. Similar to the other abdominal muscles, external oblique myofascial trigger points can refer pain anywhere locally throughout the abdominal region. This pain is often exacerbated during the menstrual cycle.

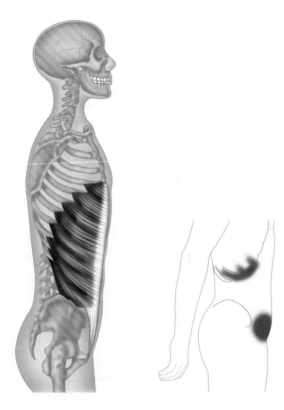

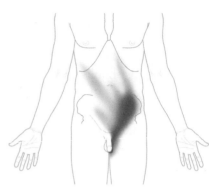

Lateral lower abdominal wall

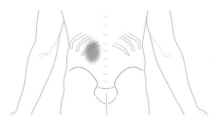

Belch button, posterior lower abdominal wall

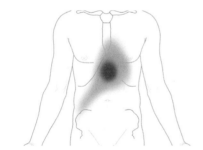

Abdominal oblique TrP referral pattern can vary considerably from patient to patient

Practitioner Guidelines
Patient positioning
This muscle can be needled either supine, as shown, or side-lying, as many fibers are located posteriorly.

Needle type
Use 0.25 to 0.30 mm × 30 mm needle.

Needling directions
A tangential approach is required for treating these myofascial trigger points, moving the needle in a lateral to medial direction and a superior to inferior direction.

Precautions
Take a tangential approach to needle insertion and avoid going deeper than the muscle depths. The peritoneal cavity lies deep to the abdominal musculature, and care is required to ensure correct needle depth.

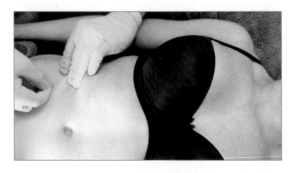

TRANSVERSUS ABDOMINIS

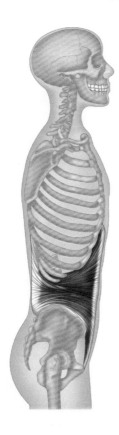

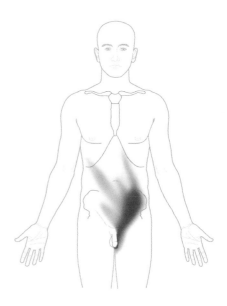

Latin, *transversus*, across, crosswise; *abdominis*, of the belly/stomach.

Origin
Costal margin, lumbar fascia, anterior two-thirds of the iliac crest, and lateral half of the inguinal ligament.

Insertion
Aponeurosis of the posterior and anterior rectus sheath, and conjoined tendon to the pubic crest and pectineal line.

Nerve
Ventral rami of thoracic nerves T7–12, ilioinguinal and iliohypogastric nerves.

Action
Supports the abdominal wall, and aids forced expiration and in raising intra-abdominal pressure. The conjoint tendon supports the posterior wall of the inguinal canal.

Kinetic Chain Comment
All abdominal muscles work on a moment-to-moment basis as we move, providing the tension required to translate forces from the lower limbs to the upper limbs. The transversus abdominis is the deepest of these muscles, and each one (right and left) wraps up the organs horizontally. Transversus abdominis fascial attachments include the lumbar vertebrae, ribcage, iliac crest, and inguinal ligament. The muscle also connects directly into the linea alba, furnishing a link between the xiphoid process, pyramidalis, and pubic bone. Transversus abdominis therefore provides essential support for the internal organs, as well as tensional support and lift for L2–3.

Myofascial Trigger Point Comment

Pain is experienced across the upper abdomen, with a focus on the xiphoid process. Patients can also experience a marked enthesitis along the inferior costal margin. Coughing is especially distressing.

Practitioner Guidelines

Patient positioning
Patient is supine or side lying.

Needle type
Use 0.25 to 0.30 mm × 30 mm needle.

Needling directions
Take a tangential approach to needle insertion and avoid going deeper than the muscle depths.

Precautions
The peritoneal cavity lies deep to the abdominal musculature, and care is required to ensure correct needle depth. With the patient in a side-lying position, the contents of the peritoneal cavity move medially, which facilitates safe needling.

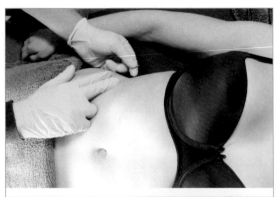

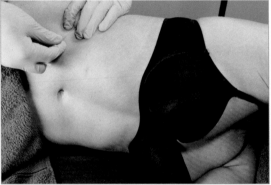

RECTUS ABDOMINIS

Latin, *rectus*, straight; *abdominis*, of the belly/stomach.

Origin
Pubic crest and symphysis pubis via two tendons separated by the linea alba.

Insertion
Costal cartilages of the fifth to seventh ribs, and xiphoid process.

Nerve
Ventral rami of thoracic nerves T5–12.

Action
With the origin fixed, the chest wall will move toward the pelvis. With the insertion fixed, the pelvis will move toward the chest.

Kinetic Chain Comment
This muscle decelerates trunk extension through eccentric action. It is worth noting that the full range of motion cannot be achieved with conventional sit-ups performed on the floor, which can contribute to muscle imbalances and neuromuscular inefficiency of the core.

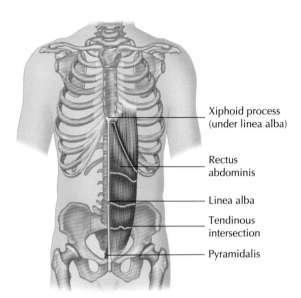

Xiphoid process
(under linea alba)

Rectus
abdominis

Linea alba

Tendinous
intersection

Pyramidalis

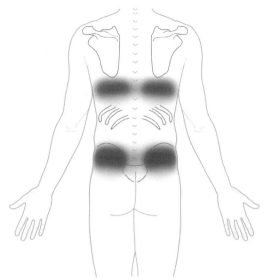

Myofascial Trigger Point Comment

Rectus abdominis has two distinct pain patterns—at the level of the xiphoid process, spreading bilaterally across the middle back—and at the level between the umbilicus and the inguinal ligament, spreading pain into the sacroiliac joint and lower back. Rectus abdominis myofascial trigger points can also cause chest pain, heartburn, belching, diarrhea, dysmenorrhea, and appendicitis (McBurney's point).

Practitioner Guidelines

Patient positioning

Patient is supine.

Needle type

Use 0.25 to 0.30 mm × 30 mm needle.

Needling directions

Direct the needle in a lateral to medial direction.

Precautions

Avoid the abdominal cavity by inserting the needle at a shallow angle, tangential to the abdominal wall.

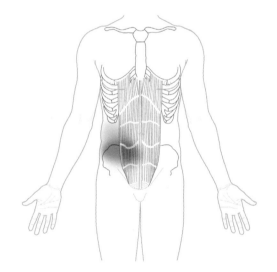

Right lateral rectus abdominis, McBurney's point

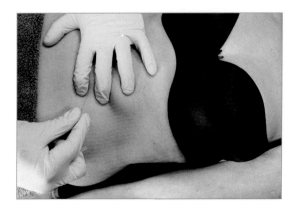

ILIOPSOAS GROUP

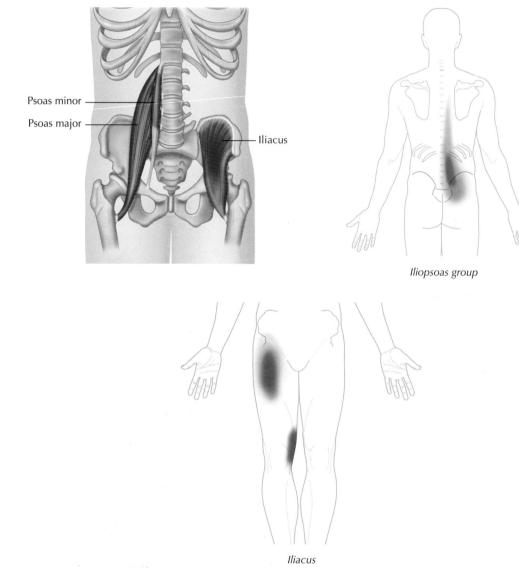

Psoas minor

Psoas major

Iliacus

Iliopsoas group

Iliacus

PSOAS MAJOR

Greek, *psoa*, muscle of the loin. **Latin**, *major*, larger.

Origin
Transverse processes of L1–5, bodies of T12–L5, and intervertebral discs below bodies of T12–L4.

Insertion
Middle surface of the lesser trochanter of the femur.

Nerve
Ventral rami of lumbar nerves L1–4.

Action
Flexes and medially rotates the hip.

Kinetic Chain Comment
Psoas major eccentrically decelerates hip extension and external rotation at the hip. This muscle is typically short, causing inhibition in the gluteal muscles, which sets up the foundation for kinetic chain neuromuscular changes and the formation of myofascial trigger points.

Myofascial Trigger Point Comment
Prolonged sitting has been identified as a significant precursor to the formation of myofascial trigger points. Myofascial trigger points form in the psoas major due to primary myofascial trigger points in related muscles of the psoas functional unit. These muscles include the rectus femoris, pectineus, sartorius, tensor fascia latae, adductors, and gracilis. Pain is felt as a vertical pattern ipsilaterally along the lumbar spine, and downward over the sacroiliac joint and gluteal region. Pain can also be present in the groin and medial thigh. Psoas pain can be mistaken for lumbago and disc pathology.

Practitioner Guidelines
Patient positioning
Patient is side lying.

Needle type
Use 0.25 to 0.30 mm × 30 mm needle.

Needling directions
Needling should occur below the level of L2, keeping the needle angled in an anterior direction.

Precautions
Check anatomical landmarks to ensure that the needle avoids the genitofemoral, lateral cutaneous, femoral, and obturator nerves, which lie on the deepest or posterior portion of this muscle.

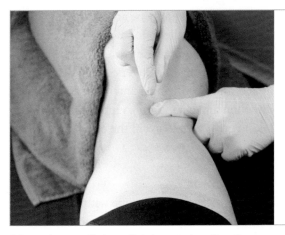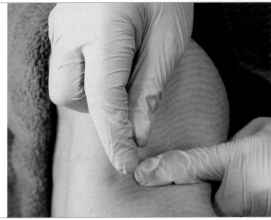

Direct the needle in a slightly anterior direction, once you have identified the taut bands.

ILIACUS

Latin, *iliacus*, relating to the loin.

Origin
Iliac fossa by means of the superior two-thirds of the crest of the ilium, iliolumbar and anterior sacroiliac ligaments, and ala of the sacrum.

Insertion
Blends with the lateral aspect of the psoas major over the pelvic rim, slightly distal to the lesser trochanter of the femur, and a few fibers merging with the joint capsule of the hip.

Nerve
Femoral nerve L2–4.

Action
With its origin fixed, the iliacus will draw the femur forward in hip flexion, adduction, and internal rotation. With the insertion fixed, and acting bilaterally, the pelvis is drawn forward, thus tilting the pelvis, with flexion at the hip but with the trunk moving, thereby increasing lumbar lordosis. Unilaterally, the iliacus will assist in lateral flexion of the trunk toward the same side.

Kinetic Chain Comment
Iliacus and psoas major (including the psoas minor if one is evident) work together to provide a deceleration of internal rotation of the femur on heel-strike and slow hip extension. Bilateral contraction of this fleshy triangular muscle provides stability to the lumbar spine. These muscles are rich in muscle spindles and are therefore prone to shorten under stress. This in turn can cause inhibition in the gluteus maximus.

Myofascial Trigger Point Comment
Myofascial trigger points can form in the gaster of iliacus and the associated psoas muscles, referring pain across the lower back and down into the buttock, anterior thigh, and groin. Difficulty breathing and urinating are often reported.

Practitioner Guidelines
Patient positioning
The patient in a side-lying (lateral recumbent) position will ensure that the therapist avoids the abdominal contents.

Needle type
Use 0.25 to 0.30 mm × 30 to 50 mm needle.

Needling directions
This muscle must only be accessed by allowing the needle to follow the path of the anterior ilium below the crest. Direct the needle between your fingers, as shown in the image, and needle in an anterior to posterior direction and a superior to inferior direction, taking great care to avoid the abdominal content.

Precautions
Only perform this technique with the patient in the lateral recumbent position, to encourage medial movement of the abdominal content.

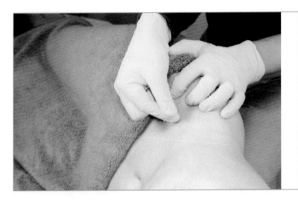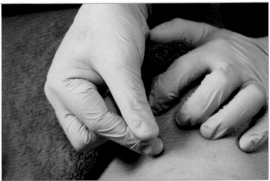

PSOAS MINOR

Greek, *psoa*, muscle of the loin. **Latin**, *minor*, smaller.

Origin
Bodies of T12 and L1 and intervening intervertebral disc.

Insertion
Fascia over the psoas major and iliacus.

Nerve
Anterior primary rami of L1, L2.

Action
Weak flexor of the trunk.

Kinetic Chain Comment
This muscle is present in only 50–60% of the population. Because of its unique relationship connecting the upper body and lower limb, any problems in this muscle result in full-body kinetic chain adaptations and distortions. Areas of pain can include the neck, lower back, knee, and foot.

Myofascial Trigger Point Comment
A possible symptom of myofascial trigger points in this muscle is a posteriorly tilted pelvis, which causes a flat-back posture and compressed intervertebral discs. Lower back pain is the classical referral pattern, but pain can also be referred into the groin and thigh.

Practitioner Guidelines
Patient positioning
Patient is side lying (lateral recumbent position).

Needle type
Use 0.25 to 0.30 mm × 30 mm needle.

Needling directions
Needling should occur below the level of L2, keeping the needle angled in an anterior direction.

Precautions
Check anatomical landmarks to ensure that the needle avoids the genitofemoral, lateral cutaneous, femoral, and obturator nerves, which lie on the deepest or posterior portion of this muscle.

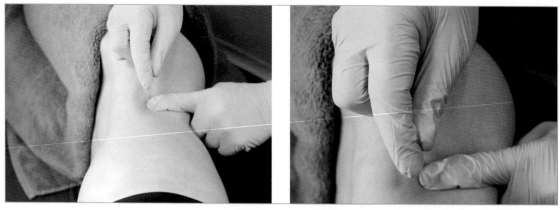

Direct the needle in a slightly anterior direction, once you have identified the taut bands.

QUADRATUS LUMBORUM

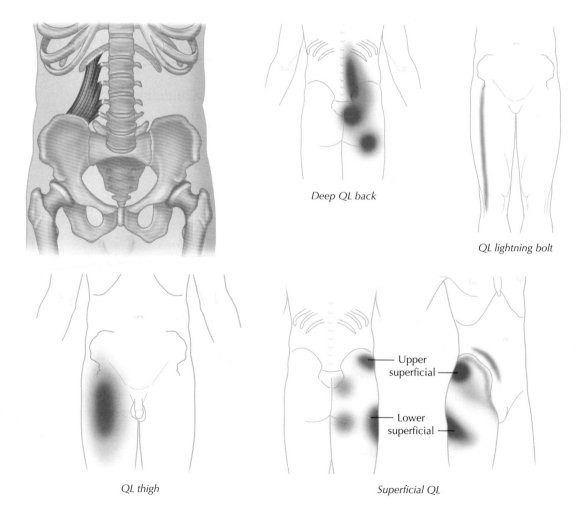

Deep QL back

QL lightning bolt

QL thigh

Upper superficial

Lower superficial

Superficial QL

Latin, *quadratus*, squared; *lumborum*, of the loins.

Origin
Inferior border of the twelfth rib.

Insertion
Apices of the transverse processes of L1–4, iliolumbar ligament, and posterior third of the iliac crest.

Nerve
Ventral rami of the subcostal nerve and upper three or four lumbar nerves T12, L1–3.

Action
Fixes the twelfth rib during respiration and laterally flexes the trunk.

Kinetic Chain Comment
A short quadratus lumborum leads to a functional short leg on the same side. This in turn leads to muscle adaptations, whereby the contralateral adductors may shorten in an effort to pull the femur more posteriorly into the acetabulum. This can create the look of a short leg on the contralateral side and cause subluxation at the pubic symphysis and sacroiliac joint. Kinetic chain problems continue both up and down the chain.

Myofascial Trigger Point Comment
Pain is experienced at the sacroiliac joint and into the gluteal muscles and the hip. Referred pain in the anterior thigh and groin can be very painful. Fear of coughing or sneezing because of intolerable pain in the lower back is common. As a result of pain on the affected side there may be difficulty sleeping.

Myofascial trigger points in the quadratus lumborum can cause the hip to hike, which can lead to a scoliosis and subsequently an anatomical short leg.

Practitioner Guidelines
Patient positioning
Patient is side lying (lateral recumbent position), with the use of bolsters to ensure patient comfort.

Needle type
Use 0.25 to 0.30 mm × 30 to 50 mm needle.

Needling directions
Needle in a medial to lateral direction, posterior to the mid-frontal plane.

Precautions
Carefully needle below L2 to avoid bringing the needle into the peritoneal cavity or the kidney. Palpate the quadratus lumborum on contraction to confirm the location of this deep muscle and assist the patient in returning the lower limb to the table following active contraction. Work slowly while checking and rechecking your anatomical landmarks.

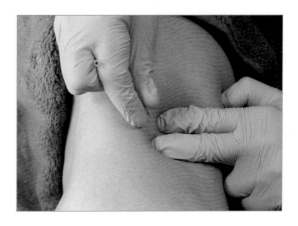

Muscles of the Shoulder and Upper Arm

TRAPEZIUS

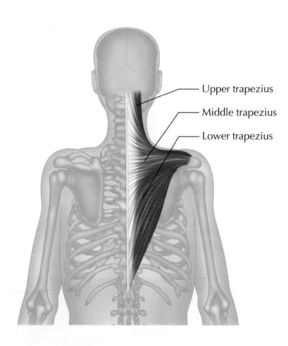

Upper trapezius
Middle trapezius
Lower trapezius

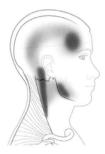

The referral pattern may be entire or in part, and usually results from TrPs in the most vertical upper trapezius fibers, occurring along the side of the neck between the collarbone attachment and the occipital attachment

Greek, *trapezoeides*, table shaped.

Origin
Medial third superior nuchal line, ligamentum nuchae, and spinous processes and supraspinous ligaments to T12.

Insertion
Upper fibers: Lateral third of the posterior border of the clavicle.
Lower fibers: Medial acromion, and superior lip of the spine of the scapula to the deltoid tubercle.

Nerve
Motor supply: Accessory XI nerve.
Sensory supply (proprioception): Ventral ramus of cervical nerves C2–4.

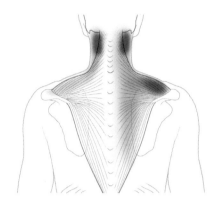

The referral pattern on the left of this figure is from TrPs found in the left most horizontal upper trapezius muscle fibers. The pattern on the right side is usually from TrPs found in the right lower trapezius, between the shoulder blade and the spine, fairly close to the shoulder blade

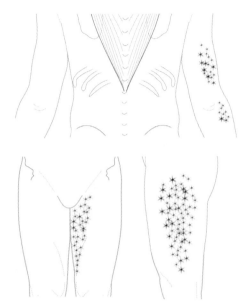

These figures represent patterns of gooseflesh rather than pain and vary with individuals. The TrPs producing them are often found in an oval trigger area above the upper inside edge of the shoulder blade triangle. Another area of TrPs can occur at the outer attachment area of the upper trapezius. TrPs in this area cause local pain

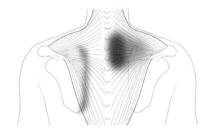

The referral pattern on the left side of this figure is usually from TrPs found in the left side, in the upper top corner attachment of the muscle covering the shoulder blade. The pattern on the right side of this figure is usually from TrPs found to the inside of the worst pain (deepest red) in the middle horizontal fibers of middle trapezius

Action

Laterally rotates, elevates, and retracts the scapula. Extends and laterally flexes the neck if the scapula is fixed.

Kinetic Chain Comment

As the trapezius is an important neck muscle, any spastic activity in the sternocleidomastoid, suboccipitals, scalenes, longus colli, levator scapulae, or many other muscles will affect its status. Many people hold emotional tension in the upper trapezius. The upper portion decelerates the head, the middle portion decelerates protraction, and the lower portion decelerates shoulder elevation.

Myofascial Trigger Point Comment

Myofascial trigger points here lead to tension headaches, with sharp pain felt in the temporal bone and into the masseter, behind the eye and ear (on the same side), and along the side of the neck. Occasionally, pain will travel to the back of the head, and a burning pain will be experienced down into the vertebral side of the scapula and middle back. Trapezius l myofascial trigger points can cause loss of balance and dizziness. Myofascial trigger points in this muscle are often mistaken for disc pathologies, neuralgia, spinal stenosis, shoulder bursitis, or arthritis.

Practitioner Guidelines

Patient positioning
Patient is either supine or prone.

Needle type
Use 0.25 to 0.30 mm × 30 mm needle.

Needling directions
Needle in a lateral to medial direction, staying well above the apex of the lung and posterior to the brachial plexus.

Precautions
Avoid the lung by holding the upper trapezius between the fingers and thumb, as shown in the image.

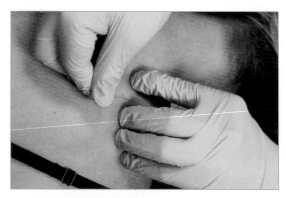

Middle trapezius, prone.

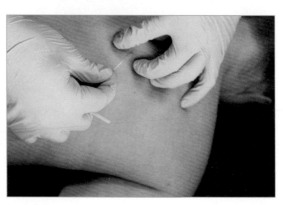

Lower trapezius, prone.

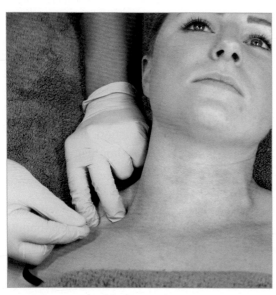

Upper trapezius, supine.

RHOMBOIDS

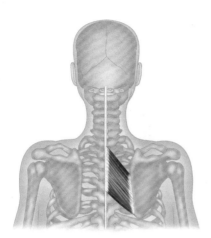

Rhomboid major

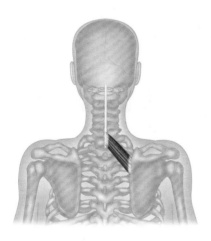

Rhomboid minor

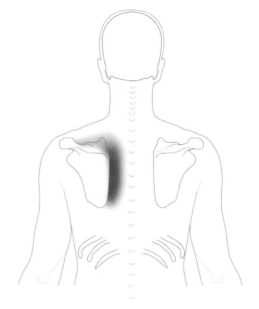

TrPs in the rhomboid major and minor and associated attachments have similar referral patterns

Greek, *rhomboeides*, parallelogram shaped, with only opposite sides and angles equal.

Origin
Spines of C7–T5 and supraspinous ligaments.

Insertion
Lower half of the posteromedial border of the scapula, from the root of the inferior angle to the upper part of the triangular area at the base of the scapular spine.

Nerve
Dorsal scapular nerve C4, C5.

Action
Retracts the scapula. Adducts, elevates, and internally rotates the scapula.

Kinetic Chain Comment
A hypertonic rhomboid will have a marked effect on the positioning of the scapula by lifting and retracting it. This will consequently inhibit the neural status of the serratus anterior, in turn affecting the external oblique, and so on along the chain. Force couple actions will be out of sequence, setting up the ideal environment for strain and overuse injury. When the serratus anterior is hypertonic, the rhomboids become inhibited, and the scapula will sit wide and drop.

Myofascial Trigger Point Comment

Pain is experienced around the vertebral border of the scapula, especially at night when at rest. The scalenes are primary sponsors of referred pain in this area and are worth treating when patients present with this pain pattern.

Practitioner Guidelines

Patient positioning
Patient is prone.

Needle type
Use 0.25 to 0.30 mm × 30 mm needle.

Needling directions
Direct the needle over the rib in a tangential manner, in an inferior to superior direction.

Precautions
There is a risk of lung penetration with all muscles covering the ribs. Ensure that the costal bone is located by placing a finger either side in the intercostal space and direct the needle onto the rib. A hypertonic rhomboid will have a marked effect on the positioning of the scapula by lifting and retracting it.

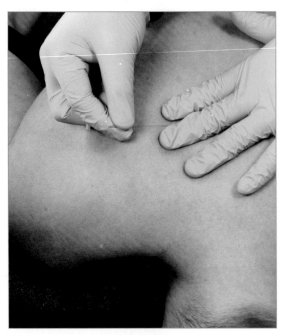

Ensure that the needle is placed over a rib.

PECTORALIS MINOR

Latin, *pectoralis*, relating to the chest; *minor*, smaller.

Origin
Third, fourth, and fifth ribs.

Insertion
Medial and upper surface of the coracoid process of the scapula.

Nerve
Medial pectoral nerve, with fibers from a communicating branch of lateral pectoral nerve C6–8, T1.

Action
Elevates the ribs if the scapula is fixed, protracts the scapula (assists the serratus anterior), and stiffens to support abduction and flexion at the shoulder joint.

Kinetic Chain Comment
Pectoralis minor provides the tension to protract the scapula against the posterior ribcage, providing a relationship with the axial skeleton so that some movement can efficiently occur at the glenohumeral joint, e.g., lateral arm raise.

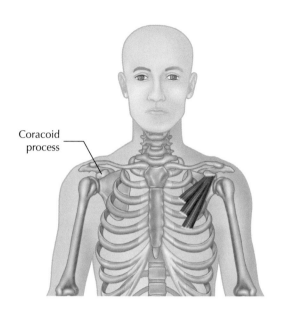

Coracoid process

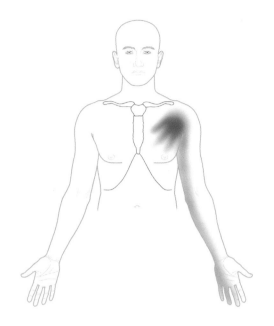

Myofascial Trigger Point Comment

Anterior chest pain is reported, with referred pain down the medial side of the arm and extending into the third to fifth digits. This pain can be mistaken for signs of heart disease but is most often mistaken for carpal tunnel syndrome because of restricted blood vessels and compressed nerves. Pectoralis minor is frequently a part of a double-crush (with the scalenes) or treble-crush problem, where all the muscles involved must be cleared of myofascial trigger points before homeostasis is restored.

Practitioner Guidelines

Patient positioning

Patient is supine.

Needle type

Use 0.25 to 0.30 mm × 30 mm needle.

Needling directions

Pectoralis minor can vary from being a very meaty muscle to being nothing short of a membrane. The coracoid process must be identified so that the needle can be directed in an inferior direction to avoid the brachial plexus.

Precautions

Placing the fingers in the intercostal space and securing the needle over the rib will ensure that the needle does not penetrate the lung.

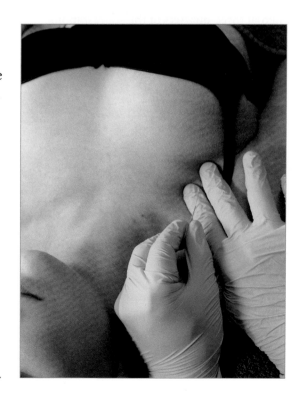

SUPRASPINATUS

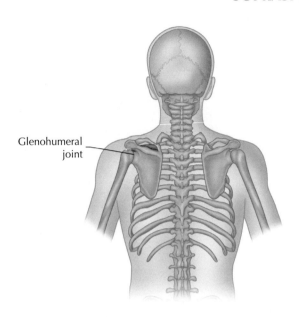

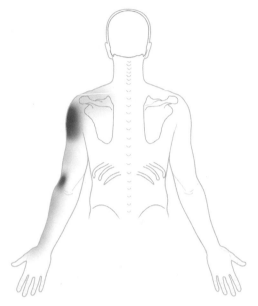

Referral pattern from the upper supraspinatus and attachment areas

Latin, *supra*, above; *spina*, spine.

Origin
Medial three-quarters of the supraspinous fossa of the scapula, and upper surface of the spine (bipennate).

Insertion
Superior facet on the greater tuberosity of the humerus, and capsule of the shoulder joint.

Nerve
Suprascapular nerve C5, C6.

Action
Abducts the arm, weak external rotator, and stabilizes the glenohumeral joint.

Kinetic Chain Comment
Supraspinatus works in conjunction with the deltoid to produce abduction at the glenohumeral joint. Because of its insertion superiorly onto the greater

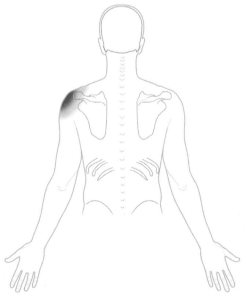

This referral pattern is from TrPs in the area of the supraspinatus tendon attachment to the glenohumeral joint

tuberosity, the muscle pulls the humeral head into the glenohumeral joint, thereby providing the stability needed while the deltoid (pulling halfway down the humerus) abducts the arm.

Myofascial Trigger Point Comment

Deep pain is reported in the lateral shoulder, forearm, and wrist. Radiating pain into the lateral epicondyle can lead to a misdiagnosis of tennis elbow (lateral epicondylitis), while the shoulder pain can be mistaken for bursitis. Difficulty combing the hair or raising the arm in flexion are signs of the presence of myofascial trigger points.

Practitioner Guidelines

Patient positioning
Patient is prone or side lying on the uninvolved shoulder.

Needle type
Use 0.25 to 0.30 mm × 30 mm needle.

Needling directions
The needle must be directed through the upper trapezius above the spine of the scapula. A tangential angle is necessary to ensure complete safety and avoid needling a fenestration in the frontal plane.

Precautions
Locate the spine of the scapula and use a shallow angle of needle insertion above the spine.

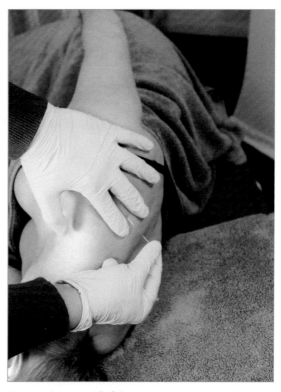

Supraspinatus, side lying.

INFRASPINATUS

Latin, *infra*, below; *spina*, spine.

Origin

Medial three-quarters of the infraspinous fossa of the scapula, and fibrous intermuscular septa.

Insertion

Middle facet of the greater tuberosity of the humerus, and capsule of the shoulder joint.

Nerve

Suprascapular nerve C5, C6.

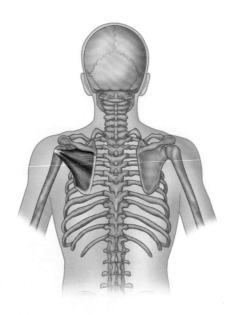

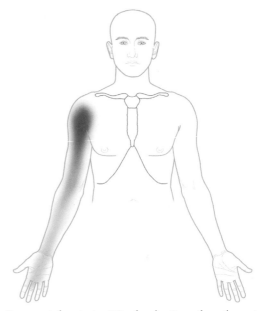

Common infraspinatus TrP referral patterns from the main portion of the muscle

Action

Laterally rotates the arm and stabilizes the shoulder joint.

Kinetic Chain Comment

Infraspinatus is an important muscle in scapula positioning because it decelerates internal rotation and shoulder flexion. Like all the rotator cuff (SITS) muscles, infraspinatus relies on an efficient core (lumbopelvic-hip complex) to translate forces needed from the lower limbs to the upper limbs.

Myofascial Trigger Point Comment

Deep shoulder joint pain is felt, as well as pain in the biceps brachii and down the side of the shoulder, radiating as far as the thumb. Severe pain in the anterior deltoid and bicipital groove are a common aspect of these myofascial trigger points, with pain also experienced in the posterior neck. Combined with other SITS muscles, these myofascial trigger points can cause symptoms mistaken for adhesive capsulitis (frozen shoulder syndrome).

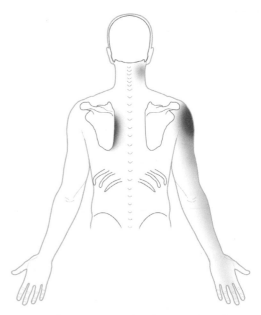

Common infraspinatus TrP referral patterns from the main portion of the muscle. TrPs in the attachment tendon of the infraspinatus cause a referral pattern along the interior shoulder blade edge, adjacent to and sometimes including the area of the TrP

Practitioner Guidelines
Patient positioning
Patient is prone or side lying on the uninvolved shoulder.

Needle type
Use 0.25 to 0.30 mm × 30 mm needle.

Needling directions
A tangential angle is necessary to ensure complete safety in the case of a fenestration. Needle in a medial to lateral direction, or—in the inferior portion—in an inferomedial to superolateral direction.

Precautions
Locate the spine of the scapula and use a shallow angle of needle insertion below the spine.

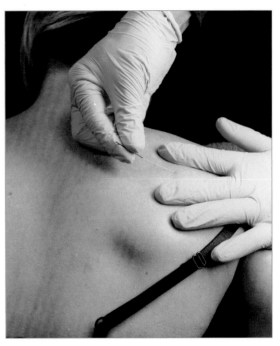

Infraspinatus, prone.

TERES MINOR

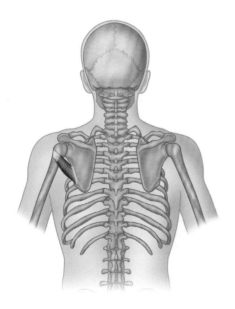

Latin, *teres*, rounded, finely shaped; *minor*, smaller.

Origin
Middle third of the lateral border of the scapula, above the teres major.

Insertion
Inferior facet of the greater tuberosity of the humerus (below infraspinatus) and capsule of the shoulder joint.

Nerve
Axillary nerve C5, C6 (from posterior cord of the brachial plexus).

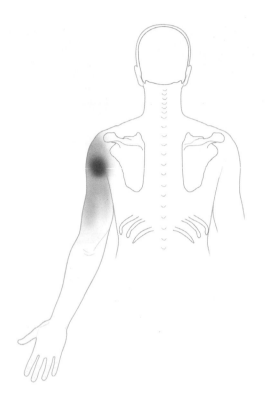

Action

Laterally rotates the arm and stabilizes the shoulder joint.

Kinetic Chain Comment

Teres minor decelerates internal rotation of the shoulder joint. Inhibition in this muscle due to short/spastic subscapularis, latissimus dorsi, teres major, and pectoralis major sets up the ideal conditions for repetitive stress in sports, such as swimming and rugby, and in any activity involving acceleration through internal/external rotation and flexion/extension of the shoulder complex.

Myofascial Trigger Point Comment

Numbness or tingling will be felt in the fourth and fifth digits of the same arm, as well as pain in the posterior shoulder at the greater tuberosity. Teres minor myofascial trigger points are often sponsored by the subscapularis.

Practitioner Guidelines

Patient positioning
Patient is prone or side lying on the uninvolved shoulder.

Needle type
Use 0.25 to 0.30 mm × 30 mm needle.

Needling directions
The pleural space is avoided by needling in a posterior medial to anterior lateral direction while holding the target fibers between the fingers and thumb, as shown in the image.

Precautions
Locate the humeral border of the scapula and needle away from this border.

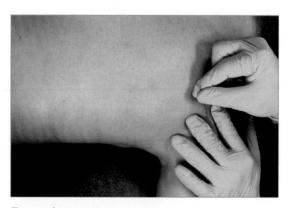

Teres minor, prone.

SUBSCAPULARIS

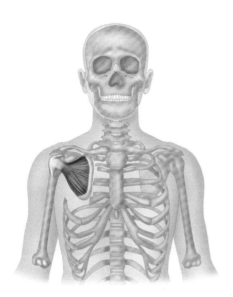

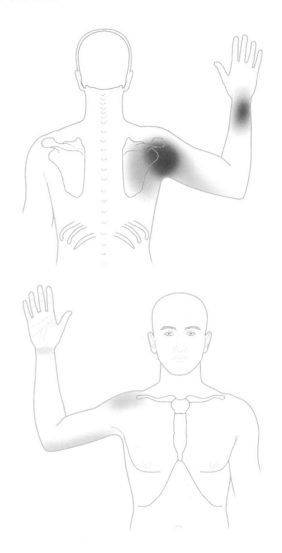

Latin, *sub*, under; *scapular*, relating to the shoulder blade.

Origin
Medial two-thirds of the subscapular fossa.

Insertion
Lesser tuberosity of the humerus, upper medial lip of the bicipital groove, and capsule of the shoulder joint.

Nerve
Upper and lower subscapular nerve C5, C6 (from posterior cord of the brachial plexus).

Action
Medially rotates the arm and stabilizes the shoulder joint.

Kinetic Chain Comment
Subscapularis eccentrically decelerates external rotation of the glenohumeral joint. This muscle has proved itself time and again to be worthy of special treatment focus in frozen shoulder and carpal tunnel syndrome complaints.

Myofascial Trigger Point Comment

Deep pain is felt in the posterior shoulder and wrist. Pain can radiate down the front of the arm. Spot tenderness on the lesser tuberosity of the humerus is common. Subscapularis myofascial trigger points are often mistaken for bursitis, adhesive capsulitis, bicipital tendinitis, arthritis, and rotator cuff injury. Pain and stiffness are a result of myofascial trigger points in the subscapularis.

Practitioner Guidelines

Patient positioning

Patient is either prone, with the upper limb in a hammerlock position, or supine, with the upper limb in flexion.

Needle type

Use 0.25 to 0.30 mm × 30 mm needle.

Needling directions

With the patient's scapula in a winged position (photograph a), the therapist can direct the needle above and parallel to the costal bones, thereby avoiding the risk of a pneumothorax.

The therapist can distract the scapula laterally (photograph b). With the patient's upper limb in flexion, the latter aspect of subscapularis is accessed by directing the needle toward the anterior surface of the scapula.

Precautions

Avoid the lungs by keeping the needle directed slightly upward or posterior toward the posterior surface of the scapula.

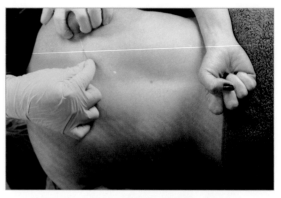

a) Patient is prone, with the upper limb in a hammerlock position to allow access to the subscapularis. Needle toward the anterior surface of the scapula.

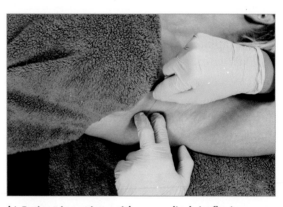

b) Patient is supine, with upper limb in flexion.

TERES MAJOR

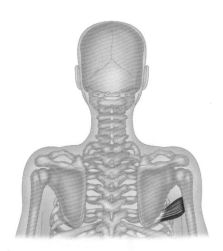

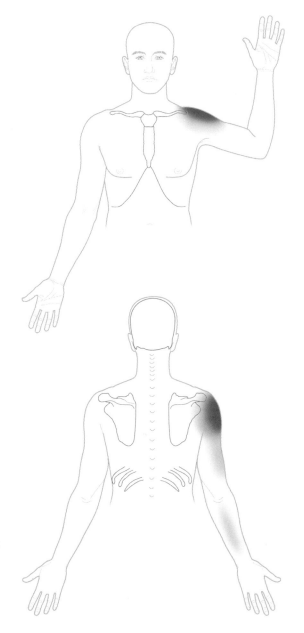

Latin, *teres*, rounded, finely shaped; *major*, larger.

Origin
Dorsal humeral surface of the inferior angle of the scapula, at the level of the lower third portion.

Insertion
Muscle fibers adhere to the fascia of the latissimus dorsi, rising up to attach to the crest of the intertubercular groove.

Nerve
Lower subscapular nerve C5–7 (from posterior cord of the brachial plexus).

Action
This muscle is affectionately known as the "little helper" of "latissimus dorsi". It medially rotates, extends, and adducts the humerus at the glenohumeral joint.

Kinetic Chain Comment
Teres major helps to eccentrically decelerate flexion, abduction, and external rotation of the humerus.

Myofascial Trigger Point Comment

Pain is experienced in the posterior deltoid.

Practitioner Guidelines

Patient positioning

Patient is prone or side lying on the uninvolved shoulder.

Needle type

Use 0.25 to 0.30 mm × 30 mm needle.

Needling directions

Teres major is located on the inferior humeral border of the scapula, deep to the latissimus dorsi. Hold the target tissues between the fingers and thumb, as shown in the image, and direct the needle in a posterior to anterior direction, parallel to the ribcage.

Precautions

Avoid the inter-pleural space.

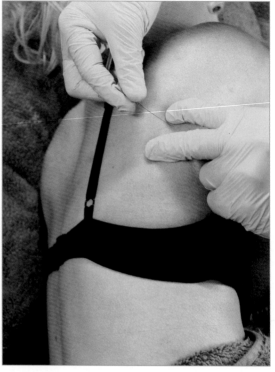

Teres major, side lying (unaffected side).

SERRATUS ANTERIOR

Latin, *serratus*, serrated; *anterior*, at the front.

Origin

Upper eight ribs and anterior intercostal membranes from the midclavicular line. Lower four interdigitate with the external oblique.

Insertion

Inner medial border of the scapula. Slips from ribs 1 and 2: upper angle; 3 and 4: length of the costal surface; 5 to 8: inferior angle.

Nerve

Long thoracic nerve C5–8 (from roots). Slips from ribs 1 and 2: C5; 3 and 4: C6; 5 to 8: C7/8.

Action

Laterally rotates and protracts scapula.

Kinetic Chain Comment

Serratus anterior eccentrically decelerates adduction and medial rotation of the inferior angle of the scapula. Actions will change, depending on the origin or insertion being fixed. With the arm static, movement occurs at the

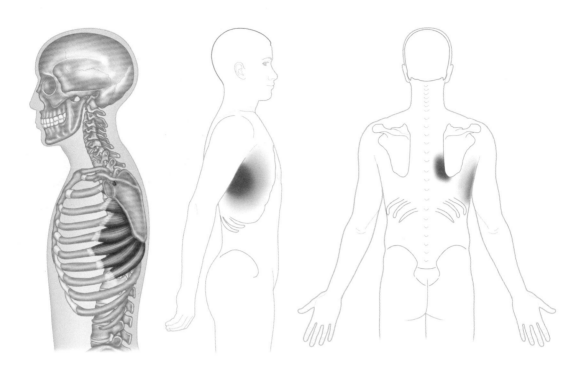

ribcage, accelerating or decelerating the ribs as required, e.g., forced exhalation.

Myofascial Trigger Point Comment

Pain will be experienced on the side of the ribcage, travelling into the armpit and posteriorly to the medial aspect of the inferior angle of the scapula. Pain is often mistaken for C8 nerve problems, as pain is referred down the inside of the arm into the palm, fifth digit (little finger), and fourth digit. As this muscle has many digitations, careful assessment is required to locate active central myofascial trigger points.

Practitioner Guidelines

Patient positioning

Patient is prone or side lying on the uninvolved shoulder.

Needle type

Use 0.25 to 0.30 mm × 30 mm needle.

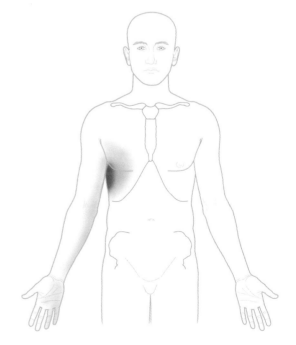

Needling directions

A tangential angle is necessary to ensure complete safety—in this case, to avoid the intercostal space. Needle above the rib, keeping a finger either side of the rib to help orientate your needle direction.

Precautions

As always, avoid any possibility of penetrating the lung.

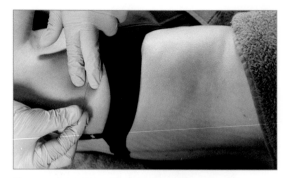

Serratus anterior, side lying (unaffected side).

LEVATOR SCAPULAE

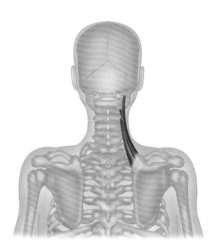
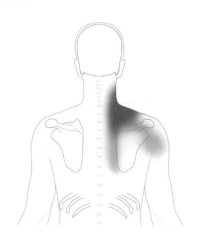

Latin, *levare*, to lift; *scapulae*, of the shoulder blade.

Origin

Posterior tubercles of the transverse processes of C1–4.

Insertion

Upper part of the medial border of the scapula.

Nerve

Dorsal scapular nerve C4, C5, and cervical nerve C3, C4.

Action

Elevates the medial border of the scapula.

Kinetic Chain Comment

Levator scapulae acts eccentrically to decelerate the downward forces created by the lower fibers of the trapezius and serratus anterior and decelerates contralateral side flexion in the cervical spine.

Myofascial Trigger Point Comment

Almost all neck pain will have myofascial trigger point contributions, and this muscle is commonly involved. Pain will be experienced at the angle of the neck from the superior angle, making its way down to the medial aspect of the inferior angle, with spillover all the way along the medial border of the scapula. Patients often report a stiff neck and reduced range of motion.

Practitioner Guidelines

Patient positioning
Patient is prone in a hammerlock position.

Needle type
Use 0.25 to 0.30 mm × 30 mm needle.

Needling directions
As shown in the image, the therapist can apply a pincer grip to the targeted fibers and inserts the needle in an inferior to superior direction. The muscle fibers are lifted away from the ribcage, ensuring that there is no risk of needling the intercostal space or causing a pneumothorax.

Precautions
Avoid directing the needle into the intercostal space.

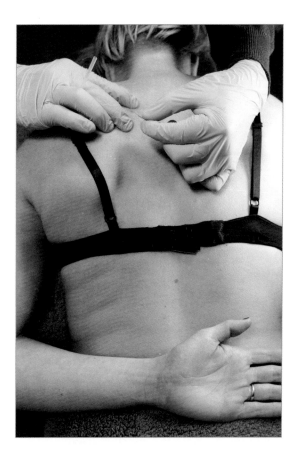

PECTORALIS MAJOR

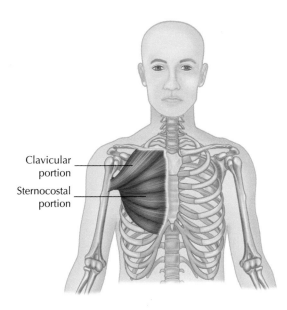

Clavicular portion

Sternocostal portion

Latin, *pectoralis*, relating to the chest; *major*, larger.

Origin
Medial half of the anterior surface of the clavicle, anterior surface of the manubrium and sternum, and cartilage of the ribs (1–6).

Insertion
By means of a laminated tendon into the lateral crest of the intertubercular groove of the humerus.

Nerve
Medial nerve C6–8, T1.

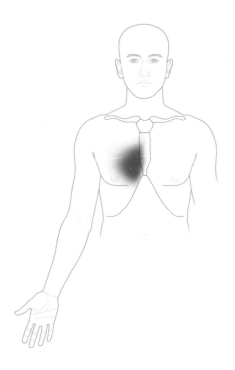

Pain from these myofascial trigger points can also be felt as interscapular and subscapular pain. Restricted abduction will be evident.

Practitioner Guidelines

Patient positioning
Patient is supine, with the upper limb abducted.

Needle type
Use 0.25 to 0.30 mm × 30 mm needle.

Needling directions
Avoid needling breast tissue. This muscle can be grasped between the fingers and thumb, lifting it off the chest wall. Direct the needle into the targeted fibers, staying parallel to the ribs.

Precautions
As always, avoid any possibility of penetrating the lung.

Action

With the origin fixed, the pectoralis major will adduct and medially rotate the humerus. With the insertion fixed, the muscle can assist in breathing (forced inspiration, as it elevates the chest). It assists in shoulder stabilization during overhead movements.

Kinetic Chain Comment

This muscle eccentrically decelerates extension, horizontal abduction, external rotation, and retraction of the shoulder joint.

Myofascial Trigger Point Comment

Pectoralis major can develop multiple myofascial trigger points because of its clavicular and sternal fibers, firing pain across the anterior deltoid and down the lateral aspect of the arm into the thumb and fourth and fifth digits. A rare myofascial trigger point can mimic the symptoms of angina pectoris.

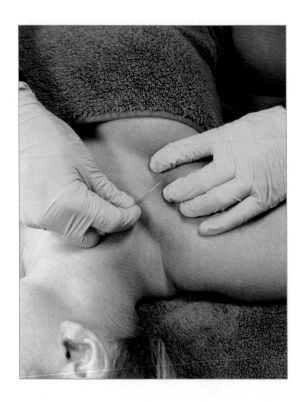

SUBCLAVIUS

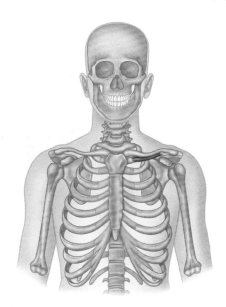

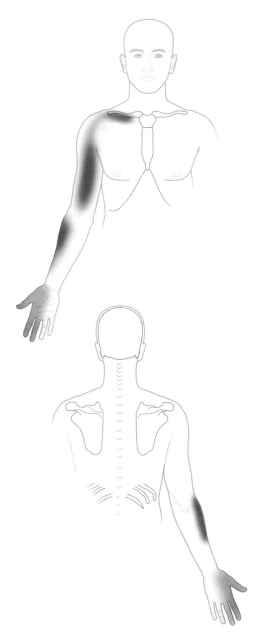

Right subclavius referral patterns

Latin, *sub*, under; *clavis*, key.

Origin
First rib, about its junction of bone and costal cartilage.

Insertion
Undersurface of the clavicle to the subclavian groove.

Nerve
Nerve to subclavius C5, C6.

Action
Pulls the clavicle toward the sternoclavicular joint.

Kinetic Chain Comment
Weak lumbopelvic-hip musculature can contribute to the formation of myofascial trigger points in subclavius. A change in position of the scapula will compromise this muscle and lead to myofascial trigger point formation.

Myofascial Trigger Point Comment
Pain is referred to the ipsilateral biceps brachii and lateral forearm. Locally, pain will be experienced just below the clavicle and may be felt as pins and needles in the

arm, shoulder, and hand. The pain typically bypasses the elbow and wrist, resulting in pain in the radial half of the hand, thumb, and middle finger.

Practitioner Guidelines

Patient positioning
Patient is supine.

Needle type
Use 0.25 to 0.30 mm × 30 mm needle.

Needling directions
Locate the inferomedial margin of the clavicle, directing the needle in an inferior lateral to superior medial direction. Avoid going any deeper than the muscle, keeping in mind the proximity of the lungs.

Precautions
As always, avoid any possibility of penetrating the lung.

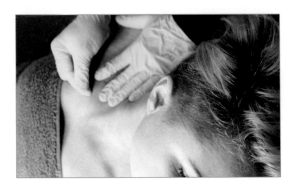

LATISSIMUS DORSI

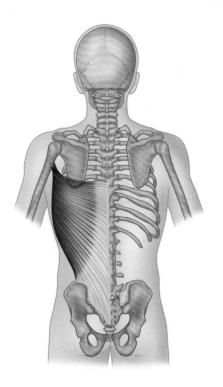

Latin, *latissimus*, widest; *dorsi*, of the back.

Origin
Spinous processes of T6–12, thoracolumbar fascia, iliac crest, and inferior three or four ribs.

Insertion
Intertubercular groove of the humerus.

Nerve
Thoracodorsal nerve C6–8.

Action
Along with its "little helper" (teres major), latissimus dorsi adducts, extends, and medially rotates the humerus in the glenohumeral joint.

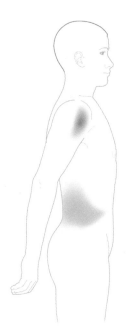

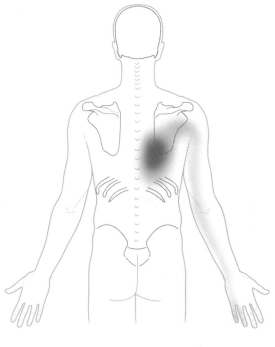

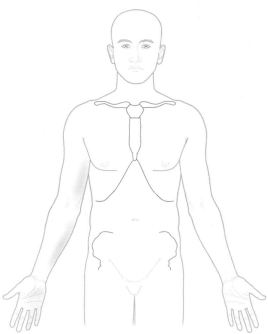

The location of the referral pattern often gives a clue to the location of the latissimus dorsi TrPs

Kinetic Chain Comment

A neuromuscular efficient core is required for the latissimus dorsi to provide the necessary forces to carry out some function at the glenohumeral joint. Neuromuscular inefficiency sets up the foundation for repetitive stress and associated "frozen shoulder"-type symptoms. The latissimus dorsi decelerates lateral rotation, flexion, and abduction of the humerus in the glenohumeral joint.

When the insertion of latissimus dorsi is fixed, the muscle plays a role in tilting the pelvis in an anterolateral direction. A bilateral contraction leads to hyperextension of the lower back, with accompanying anterior tilting of the pelvis. A muscle this size, covering so much of the posterolateral ribcage, will have an influence on diaphragmatic function. Any movement of the humerus will have an effect that extends into the thoracolumbar fascia and further down the kinetic chain.

Concerning satellite myofascial trigger points, consider the following: pectoralis major, teres major, subscapularis, triceps brachii, scalenes, upper rectus abdominis, iliocostalis, serratus anterior, serratus posterior superior and inferior, lower trapezius, and rhomboids.

Myofascial Trigger Point Comment
Latissimus dorsi generates pain in the mid-thoracic area, including the posterolateral abdominal region. Pain of an aching nature is reported in the inferior angle of the scapula and the posterior shoulder. Referred pain travels down the medial aspect of the humerus into the forearm, hand, and fingers.

Practitioner Guidelines
Patient positioning
Patient is supine, prone, or side lying on the uninvolved shoulder.

Needle type
Use 0.25 to 0.30 mm × 30 mm needle.

Needling directions
The therapist uses a pincer grip, drawing the muscle laterally. The needle is directed in an anterior to posterior direction, away from the ribcage.

Precautions
As always, avoid any possibility of penetrating the lung.

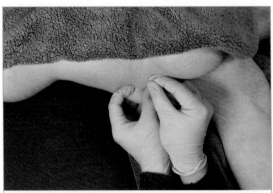

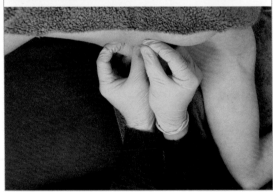

Latissimus dorsi, supine with the upper limb abducted and externally rotated.

DELTOID

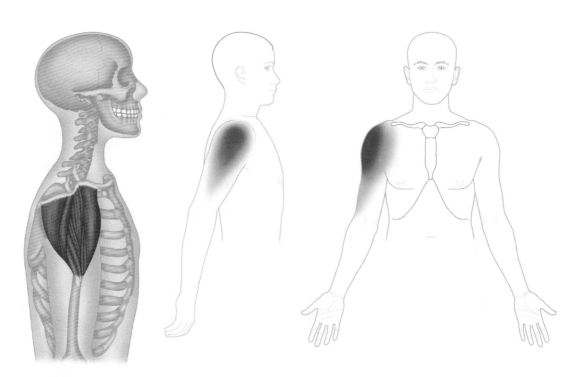

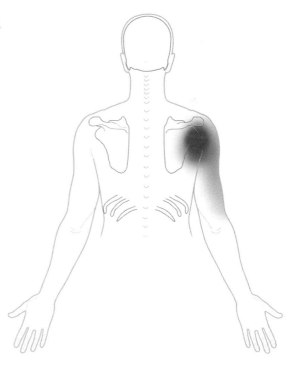

Greek, *deltoeides*, shaped like the Greek capital letter delta (Δ).

Origin
Lateral third of the clavicle, acromion, and spine of the scapula to the deltoid tubercle.

Insertion
Middle of the lateral surface of the humerus (deltoid tuberosity).

Nerve
Axillary nerve C5, C6 (from posterior cord of the brachial plexus).

Action
Abducts the arm, anterior fibers flex and medially rotate, posterior fibers extend and laterally rotate.

Kinetic Chain Comment

Deltoid—along with supraspinatus and associated rotator cuff muscles—will regularly develop myofascial trigger points as result of reduced core efficiency. Failure to translate forces from the lower body to the shoulder will result in arthrokinematic stress and the formation of active myofascial trigger points. The restoration of core neuromuscular efficiency will provide a foundation for myofascial trigger point therapy, utilizing neuromuscular therapy and medical exercise.

Myofascial Trigger Point Comment

Pain is felt as a dull ache for the most part, with increased pain on contraction of the muscle or when attempts are made to move the arm. Pain is most often mistaken for bursitis or rotator cuff injury. It is worthwhile checking the muscles that refer pain into the deltoid (SITS, pectorals, and scalenes) as the true source of deltoid pain. Deltoid myofascial trigger points are more often than not "satellite myofascial trigger points".

Practitioner Guidelines

Patient positioning

Lateral and posterior aspect myofascial trigger point dry needling is carried out with the patient in a side-lying or supine position, while the anterior fibers can be targeted in the supine position.

Needle type

Use 0.25 to 0.30 mm × 30 mm needle.

Needling directions

Using flat palpation, locate and secure the myofascial trigger point within the palpable taut band. Insert the needle and direct it into the myofascial trigger point, toward the humerus.

Precautions

No special precautions.

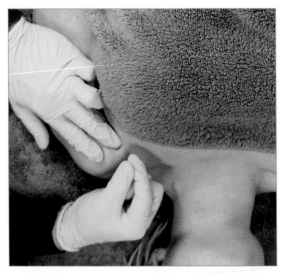

Anterior deltoid, supine.

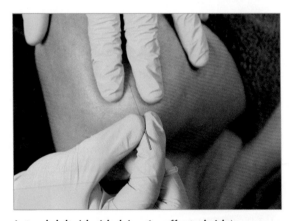

Lateral deltoid, side lying (unaffected side).

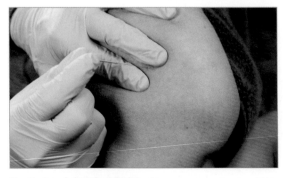

Posterior deltoid, side lying.

BICEPS BRACHII

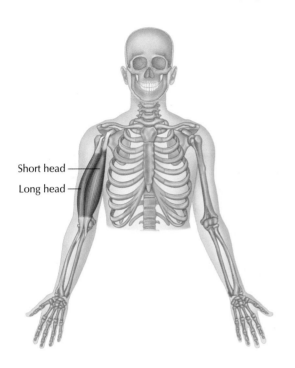

Short head —
Long head —

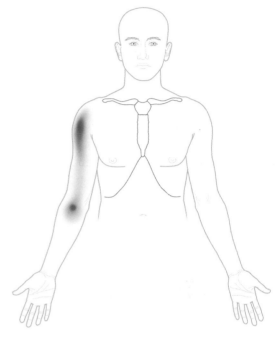

Latin, *biceps*, two-headed; *brachii*, of the arm.

Origin
Short head: A flat tendon shared with the coracobrachialis, from the apex of the coracoid process of the scapula.
Long head: Supraglenoid tubercle of the scapula, and adjacent glenoid labrum of the glenohumeral joint.

Insertion
Posterior part of the tuberosity of the radius, and aponeurosis of biceps brachii.

Nerve
Musculocutaneous nerve C5, C6

Action
With the origin of the biceps brachii fixed, flexion will occur at the elbow, initiating supination of the forearm. With the insertion

fixed, the humerus is moved toward the forearm. This muscle is also an important flexor of the shoulder joint through the action of its long head, as well as an important shoulder stabilizer.

Kinetic Chain Comment
Biceps brachii decelerates extension and pronation at the elbow and extension at the shoulder joint. It acts as a junction providing myofascial continuity between the thumb and the ribcage (especially obvious when the upper limb is abducted). The muscle plays a vital role in shoulder stability under dynamic conditions and can contract with triceps brachii to stabilize the elbow.

Myofascial Trigger Point Comment
Myofascial trigger points typically evolve in the center of the gaster and refer pain up toward the anterior deltoid and down toward the pronator teres, just distal to the

elbow joint. The neuromuscular therapy hypothesis includes weak core stability with poor neuromuscular efficiency, culminating in compensatory myofascial trigger point formation to provide additional tension.

Practitioner Guidelines

Patient positioning
Trigger point dry needling of biceps brachii is carried out with the patient in a supine position, with slight shoulder abduction and slight elbow flexion.

Needle type
Use 0.25 to 0.30 mm × 30 mm needle.

Needling directions
Using a pincer grip, locate and secure the myofascial trigger point within the palpable taut band. Insert the needle in a lateral to medial direction into the myofascial trigger point, toward or in the direction of the therapist's thumb, as shown in the image.

Precautions
Avoid the radial nerve, located on the distal lateral aspect of this muscle.

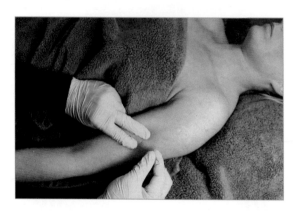

CORACOBRACHIALIS

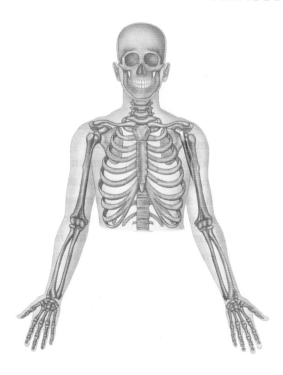

Greek, *korakoeides*, raven-like. **Latin**, *brachialis*, relating to the arm.

Origin
Coracoid process of the scapula, along with biceps brachii.

Insertion
Upper half of the medial border of the humerus.

Nerve
Musculocutaneous nerve C5–7 (from lateral cord).

Action
Flexes and weakly adducts the arm.

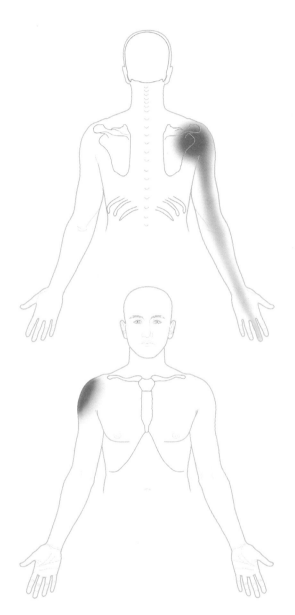

into the periosteum of the upper limb, and traveling on through the brachioradialis all the way to the radial styloid.

Myofascial Trigger Point Comment

Pain and/or numbness can be felt as far away as the posterior surface of the hand and into the middle finger. Pain can be referred to the posterior forearm, triceps brachii, and anterior deltoid.

Practitioner Guidelines

Patient positioning
Patient is supine.

Needle type
Use 0.25 to 0.30 mm × 30 mm needle.

Needling directions
The muscle is identified and needled in a superior medial to inferior lateral direction.

Precautions
The musculocutaneous nerve perforates this muscle. Other structures in its proximity include the median nerve, brachial artery, and ulnar nerve. Work slowly and look for patient feedback.

Kinetic Chain Comment

Coracobrachialis links the thoracic cage and the scapula with the arm because it shares the tendinous root onto the coracoid process with pectoralis minor. Raising the arm out into abduction, with the hand at the level of the ear, demonstrates the continuity from the pectoralis minor through the coracobrachialis

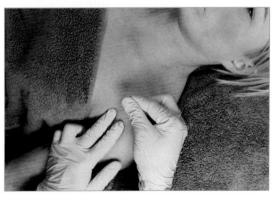

BRACHIALIS

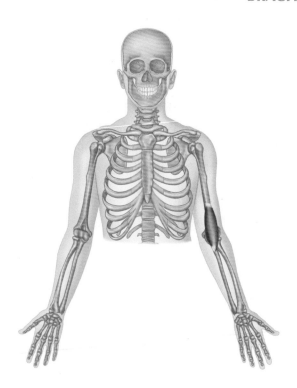

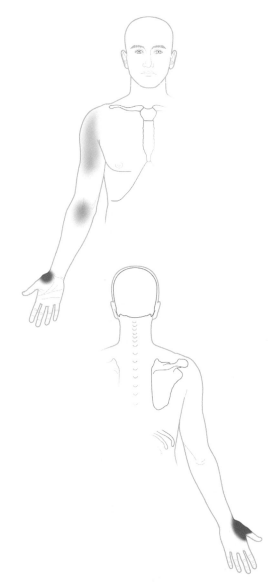

Latin, *brachialis*, relating to the arm.

Origin
Anterior lower half of the humerus, and medial and lateral intermuscular septa.

Insertion
Coronoid process and tuberosity of the ulna.

Nerve
Musculocutaneous nerve C5, C6 (from lateral cord). Also small supply from radial nerve C7.

Action
Flexes the elbow.

Kinetic Chain Comment
Brachialis is an important link muscle in the chain, connecting the thorax to the upper limb. This muscle has the potential to trap the radial nerve, resulting in numbness or other nerve-related sensations, including dysesthesia of the thumb. Myofascial trigger points could also cause such symptoms.

Myofascial Trigger Point Comment
Pain spreads to the base of the thumb, anterior deltoid, and just below the elbow joint line. Patients often complain of tingling

or numbness in the thumb and hand. These problems can be misdiagnosed as carpal tunnel syndrome.

Practitioner Guidelines
Patient positioning
Patient is supine.

Needle type
Use 0.25 to 0.30 mm × 30 mm needle.

Needling directions
The muscle is identified and needled in a lateral to medial direction to avoid the associated neurovascular structures.

Precautions
Having identified the muscle with flat palpation, needle in the septal space between the biceps brachii and triceps brachii to avoid the neurovascular structures.

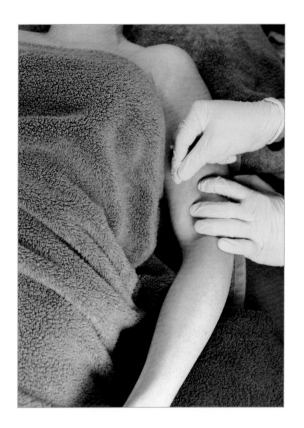

TRICEPS BRACHII

Latin, *triceps,* three-headed; *brachii,* of the arm.

Origin
Long head: Infraglenoid tubercle of the scapula.
Lateral head: Upper half of the posterior humerus (linear origin).
Medial head: Lies deep on the lower half of the posterior humerus, inferomedial to the spiral groove and both intermuscular septa.

Insertion
Posterior part of the upper surface of the olecranon process of the ulna, and posterior capsule.

Nerve
Radial nerve C6–8, T1.

Action
Extends the elbow. The long head stabilizes the shoulder joint. The medial head retracts the capsule of the elbow joint on extension.

Kinetic Chain Comment
Along with its "little helper," anconeus, triceps brachii assists deceleration of flexion at the glenohumeral joint and the elbow joint. The radial nerve can be irritated by contracture or spasm of the lateral aspect of this muscle.

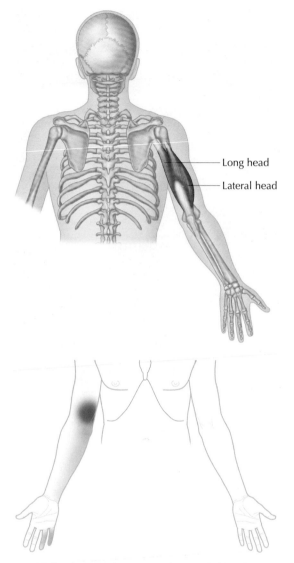

Long head
Lateral head

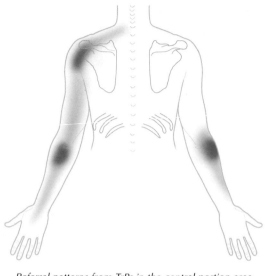

Referral patterns from TrPs in the central portion area of the left long head and from TrPs in the central portion of the right deep medial head

Referral pattern from TrPs in deep medial border of right deep medial head

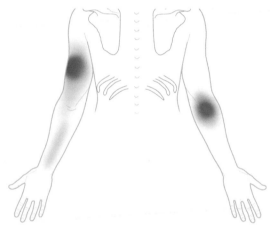

Referral pattern from TrPs in the area of the left lateral border of the left lateral head and from the right musculotendinous attachment area deep under the tendon

Myofascial Trigger Point Comment

Pain can be felt in the neck and upper trapezius. Other symptoms can lead to a misdiagnosis of pain felt in the elbow and triceps brachii as tennis or golfer's elbow.

Myofascial trigger points in this muscle make it difficult to extend the arm at the elbow. Patients complain that they cannot rest their elbow on any surface, because of the level of sensitivity and pain.

Practitioner Guidelines

Patient positioning
Patient is side lying, with the upper limb supported.

Needle type
Use 0.25 to 0.30 mm × 30 mm needle.

Needling directions
The muscle is identified and needled using a pincer grip to lift the muscle off the bone. Needle in a lateral to medial direction and an anterior to posterior direction.

Precautions
Palpate for and avoid the radial nerve, which lies in proximity to the lateral head of the triceps brachii.

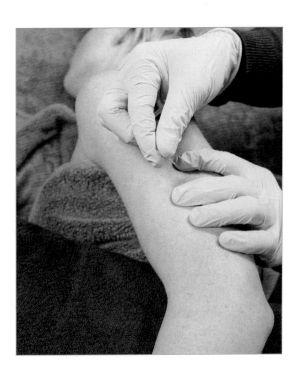

ANCONEUS

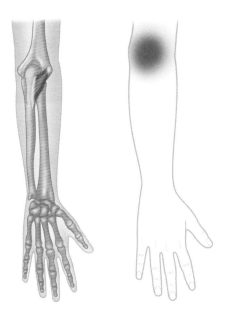

Greek, *agkon*, elbow.

Origin
Smooth surface at the lower extremity of the posterior aspect of the lateral epicondyle of the humerus.

Insertion
Lateral side of the olecranon.

Nerve
Radial nerve C7, C8.

Action
Weak extensor of the elbow and abducts the ulna in pronation.

Kinetic Chain Comment

Anconeus decelerates elbow flexion and supination. Myofascial trigger points typically evolve due to *active* myofascial trigger points in the more superior and medial muscles of the neck and shoulder. Myofascial trigger points can also evolve here because of gripping too tightly—e.g., a golf club, tennis racket, or writing pen—but reduced core strength must be considered as a causative factor.

Myofascial Trigger Point Comment

Pain from myofascial trigger points in this muscle are often mistaken for tennis elbow. Pain will be experienced when trying to flex the elbow joint and supinate the forearm.

Practitioner Guidelines

Patient positioning
Patient is side lying.

Needle type
Use 0.25 to 0.30 mm × 30 mm needle.

Needling directions
The muscle is identified and needled in a superior medial to inferior lateral direction.

Precautions
Be aware of the location of the joint space and avoid this area.

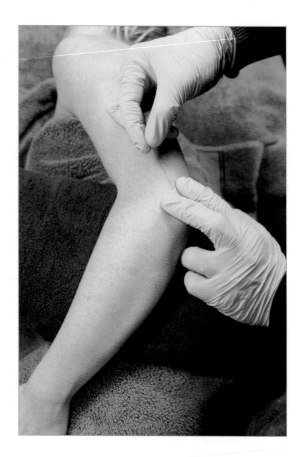

Muscles of the Forearm and Hand

PRONATOR TERES

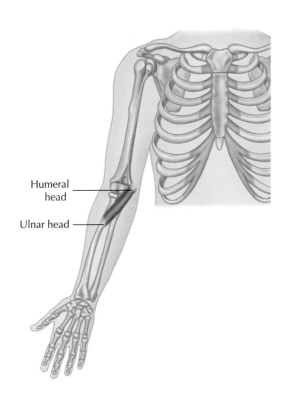

Humeral
head

Ulnar head

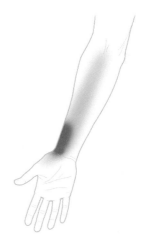

Insertion
Middle of the lateral surface of the radius.

Nerve
Median nerve C6, C7.

Action
Pronates and flexes the forearm at the elbow.

Kinetic Chain Comment
Decelerates supination and extension of the forearm at the elbow.

Latin, *pronare*, to bend forward; *teres*, rounded, finely shaped.

Origin
Medial epicondyle of the humerus, and coronoid process of the ulna.

Myofascial Trigger Point Comment

Pain is reported on the ulnar side of the forearm and at the base of the thumb. It may be difficult to turn the palm into supination with extension, without pain and stiffness. Patients have difficulty cupping the hand.

Practitioner Guidelines

Patient positioning

Patient is supine.

Needle type

Use 0.25 to 0.30 mm × 30 mm needle.

Needling directions

The muscle is identified and needled in a superior medial to inferior lateral direction.

Precautions

The median nerve, located between the two heads of this muscle, should be avoided.

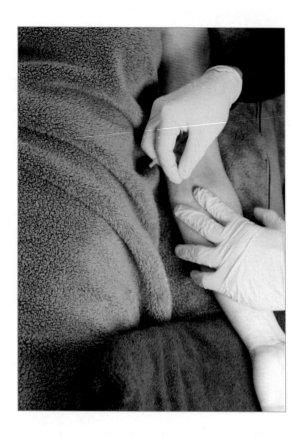

FOREARM FLEXORS

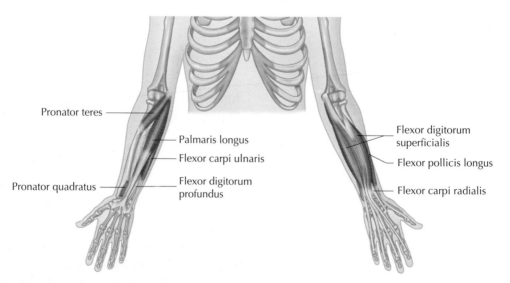

Pronator teres

Palmaris longus

Flexor carpi ulnaris

Pronator quadratus

Flexor digitorum profundus

Flexor digitorum superficialis

Flexor pollicis longus

Flexor carpi radialis

Although the extensor retinaculum is an extensor rather than a flexor, the retinacula are placed together here. TrPs in the extensor retinaculum seem to be more common in computer users. Those in the flexor retinaculum are more common in gymnasts.

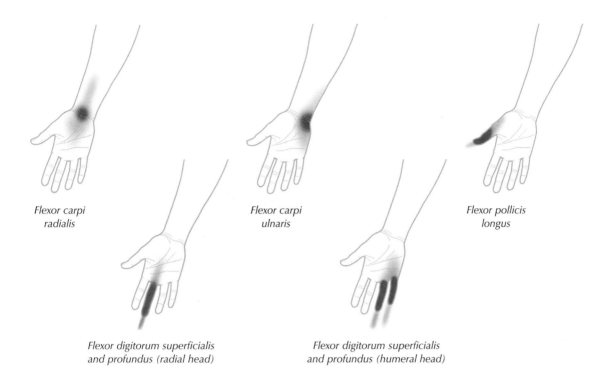

Flexor carpi radialis

Flexor carpi ulnaris

Flexor pollicis longus

Flexor digitorum superficialis and profundus (radial head)

Flexor digitorum superficialis and profundus (humeral head)

Latin, *flectere*, to bend.

Origin
Medial epicondyle of the humerus.

Insertion
Digits of the hand—carpals, metacarpals, and thumb.

Nerve
Radial and ulnar nerves.

Action
Flexion of the wrist and fingers.

Kinetic Chain Comment
A common theme in this book is the notion that the upper limb relies on forces to be translated from the lower limbs through the core, so that the arms can carry out some function. A lack of core stability will lead to these muscles developing extra stiffness in an effort to provide the forces required when communication has broken down within the kinetic chain. Habitual tasks will determine which muscles shorten and which become inhibited; typically, the forearm flexors will shorten, while the extensors will become inhibited.

Treatment of the flexors first can often yield the best results, followed by medical exercise to build extensor endurance and tone.

Myofascial Trigger Point Comment
As there are numerous muscles in this area, various pain pattern behaviors will be influenced by specific muscles. In general, these myofascial trigger points refer pain into the anterior part of the hand and lateral three fingers. Spray and stretch technique is particularly good in the treatment of these muscles and restoration of homeostasis.

Practitioner Guidelines

Patient positioning
Patient is supine.

Needle type
Use 0.25 to 0.30 mm × 30 mm needle.

Needling directions
The individual flexor muscles are identified and needled in a superior to inferior direction, using an angled motion. Needling 1–2 cm below the medial epicondyle should be done to avoid the median and ulnar nerves.

The ulnar nerve (medial side of forearm) can be clearly palpated; it pierces the two heads of the flexor carpi ulnaris and travels on the medial side of the ulna between the flexor carpi ulnaris and the deeper flexor digitorum profundus. Palpate the median nerve as it runs between flexor digitorum profundus and flexor digitorum superficialis, to enter the hand at the carpal tunnel.

Precautions
Palpate the nerves to make sure you avoid them. Working slowly and getting feedback from your patient, however, will ensure that you avoid the neurovascular structures.

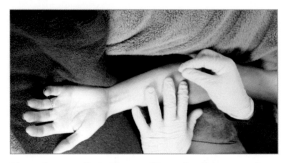

Here the needle is directed into the flexor carpi radialis. Redirect the needle to any of the forearm muscles once the myofascial trigger point has been identified.

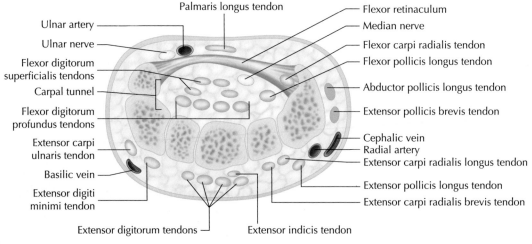

Cross-section of the wrist.

ADDUCTOR POLLICIS

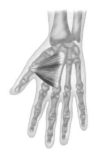
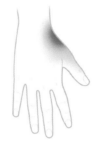
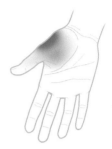

It is worth pointing out at this stage to remember which other muscles refer pain into these areas—the scalenes, brachialis, supinator, extensor carpi radialis longus, and brachioradialis. Remember to check these muscles first (in the order of most medial and superior).

Latin, *adducere,* to lead to; *pollicis,* of the thumb.

Origin
Flexor retinaculum, and tubercles of the scaphoid and trapezium.

Insertion
Lateral side of the base of the proximal phalanx of the thumb.

Nerve
Deep ulnar nerve C8, T1.

Action
Abducts the thumb and helps oppose it.

Kinetic Chain Comment
Decelerates abduction of the thumb.

Myofascial Trigger Point Comment
Aching pain is felt on the outside of the thumb and on the hand at the base of the thumb, which has a tendency to lock. Patients find it difficult to control movement of the thumb and have difficulty holding a pen. Difficulty fastening buttons or performing actions that require fine muscle control becomes evident.

Myofascial trigger point pain can be felt in the thumb web space and the thenar eminence.

Practitioner Guidelines
Patient positioning
Patient is supine, with the forearm supported.

Needle type
Use 0.14 to 0.16 mm × 15 mm needle.

Needling directions
The muscle is needled through the posterior skin surface between the thumb and the first finger.

Precautions
Fine, short needles are recommended.

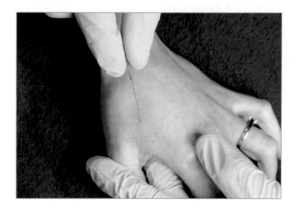

ABDUCTOR POLLICIS LONGUS

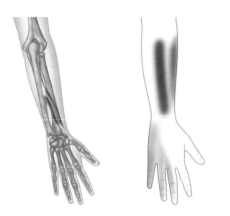

Latin, *abducere*, to lead away from; *pollicis*, of the thumb; *longus*, long.

Origin
Posterior surfaces of the ulna and the radius, and interosseous membrane.

Insertion
Base of the first metacarpal.

Nerve
Posterior interosseous nerve C6–8.

Action
Abducts and extends the thumb at the carpometacarpal joint.

Kinetic Chain Comment
Decelerates adduction of the thumb.

Myofascial Trigger Point Comment
Abductor pollicis longus is one of a number of muscles that can generate stiffness in the hand and fingers, often mistaken for arthritis. Patients have reported waking from their sleep because of cramping. As a result of inhibitory influences, the fingers and forearm lose local endurance, and fatigue sets in early on. Skilled control of the thumb reduces.

Referred pain patterns of the abductor pollicis longus resemble the C6–8 dermatomes, the superficial radial sensory nerve distribution, and are very similar to the area of pain experienced in de Quervain's tenosynovitis. Identification of abductor pollicis longus myofascial trigger points should be considered in the case of pain of the radial aspect of the wrist and thumb, especially when other neurological abnormalities or inflammatory conditions have been ruled out.

Practitioner Guidelines
Patient positioning
Patient is supine, with the forearm supported and pronated.

Needle type
Use 0.25 to 0.30 mm × 30 mm needle.

Needling directions
The muscle is identified and needled in a superior medial to inferior lateral direction.

Precautions
At this point of the forearm—needle depth is a key issue—and the interosseous membrane should be avoided. Palpate for nerves, including the branches of the radial nerve, and avoid.

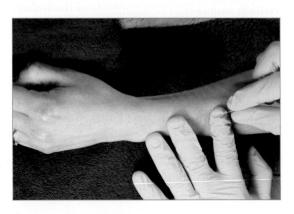

PRONATOR QUADRATUS

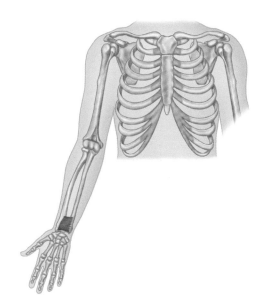

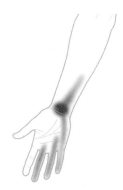

Latin, *pronare*, to bend forward; *quadratus*, squared.

Origin
Distal quarter of the shaft of the ulna.

Insertion
Distal shaft of the radius.

Nerve
Anterior interosseous from median nerve C7, C8, T1.

Action
Pronates the forearm. Deep fibers bind the radius and the ulna together.

Kinetic Chain Comment
Failure to stabilize the relationship between the radius and the ulna leads to complications along the upper limb fascial sleeve, resulting in shoulder joint and shoulder girdle/neck problems. Attempts to strengthen the forearm through increased weight training or similar will result in compounding the patient's problems. Pronator quadratus must have its myofascial trigger points dealt with before an appropriate course of physical activity with an emphasis on endurance is introduced.

Myofascial Trigger Point Comment
Two main pain patterns are observed. The most common pattern involves pain spreading both distally and proximally along the medial aspect of the forearm. In some cases, the pain area extends to the medial epicondyle proximally and the fifth digit distally. The second main pattern is pain spreading distally to the third and/or fourth digit. The pain patterns originating from the pronator quadratus resemble the C8–T1 dermatomes, and ulnar and median nerve sensory distributions. Therefore, myofascial pain of the pronator quadratus should be considered as a possible cause of pain in the medial forearm and hand, especially when other neurological abnormalities have been ruled out.

Practitioner Guidelines
Dry needling of the pronator quadratus is not recommended.
(Alternatively, positional release techniques can be used.)

ABDUCTOR POLLICIS BREVIS

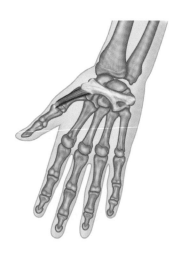

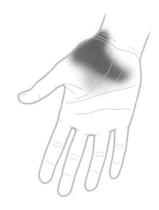

Latin, *abducere*, to lead away from; *pollicis*, of the thumb; *brevis*, short.

Origin
Flexor retinaculum, transverse carpal ligament, and tubercles of the scaphoid and trapezium.

Insertion
Lateral side of the base of the proximal phalanx of the thumb.

Nerve
Recurrent branch of median nerve C7, C8, and T1.

Action
Abducts the thumb and helps to oppose it.

Kinetic Chain Comment
Decelerates adduction of the thumb.

Myofascial Trigger Point Comment
Patients have reported a loss of grip strength. Pain and sensations are experienced in the palmar aspect of the thumb and wrist (radial side).

Practitioner Guidelines
Patient positioning
Patient is supine, with the forearm pronated.

Needle type
Use 0.25 to 0.30 mm × 30 mm needle.

Needling directions
Direct the needle from the thumb side to the little-finger side, along the posterior portion of the middle third of the radius.

Precautions
It is recommended to use a shallow angle of needle application, thus avoiding the interosseous membrane.

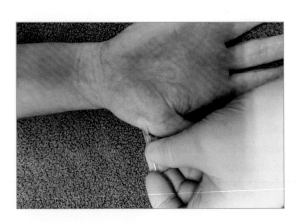

ABDUCTOR DIGITI MINIMI

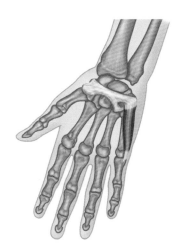

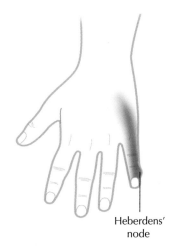

Heberdens' node

Latin, *abducere*, to lead away from; *digiti*, of the finger; *minimi*, of the smallest.

Origin
Pisiform bone, and tendon of the flexor carpi ulnaris.

Insertion
Medial side of the base of the proximal phalanx of the little finger.

Nerve
Deep branch of ulnar nerve C8 and T1.

Action
Abducts the fifth digit (little finger).

Kinetic Chain Comment
Decelerates adduction of the fifth digit.

Myofascial Trigger Point Comment
As the name of the muscle would suggest, pain and stiffness are felt in the little finger and often described as being an arthritic-type pain.

Practitioner Guidelines
Patient positioning
Patient is supine, with the forearm pronated.

Needle type
Use 0.14 to 0.16 mm × 15 mm needle.

Needling directions
Direct the needle in a medial to lateral direction, along the posterior portion of the middle third of the radius.

Precautions
The median nerve is located between the flexor digitorum superficialis and the flexor digitorum profundus and should be avoided.

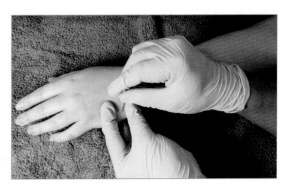

BRACHIORADIALIS

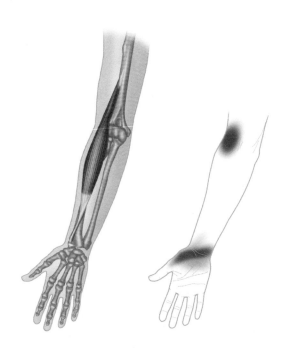

Latin, *brachium*, arm; *radius*, staff, spoke of wheel.

Origin
Proximal two-thirds of the lateral supracondylar ridge of the humerus, and lateral intermuscular septal fascia.

Insertion
Lateral surface of the distal end of the radial styloid process.

Nerve
Radial nerve C5, C6.

Action
Flexes the elbow joint and assists in pronation and supination of the forearm.

Kinetic Chain Comment
Brachioradialis is an important muscle in joining the forearm and anatomical arm, decelerating extension of the forearm at the elbow. It is a classic example of a "shunt muscle," preventing, as it does, the separation of the elbow joint during rapid movements. Baby or satellite myofascial trigger points should include the supinator, extensor carpi radialis longus, triceps brachii, and extensor digitorum.

Myofascial Trigger Point Comment
Pain is referred to the wrist and the base of the thumb in the web space. Pain is also felt at the lateral epicondyle. A full examination of all the associated muscles in the kinetic chain must be carried out.

Practitioner Guidelines
Patient positioning
Patient is supine, with slight elbow flexion and with the forearm slightly pronated or in a neutral position.

Needle type
Use 0.25 to 0.30 mm × 30 mm needle.

Needling directions

Insert the needle from the medial or lateral side of the proximal forearm and direct it toward the fingers (move the needle superior to inferior).

Precautions

Avoid needling the radial nerve, which runs close to brachioradialis over the lateral epicondyle of the humerus, through the cubital fossa. Be aware of the needle depth and direction to avoid needling your own finger.

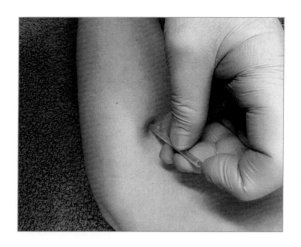

EXTENSOR CARPI RADIALIS BREVIS

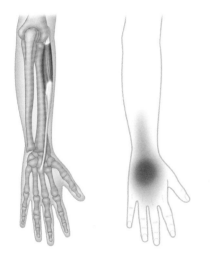

Latin, *extendere*, to extend; *carpi*, of the wrist; *radius*, staff, spoke of wheel; *brevis*, short.

Origin
Lateral epicondyle of the humerus.

Insertion
Posterior base of the third metacarpal bone.

Nerve
Radial nerve C5–8.

Action
Extends the wrist and hand and abducts the hand.

Kinetic Chain Comment
Decelerates flexion of the wrist and hand and adduction of the hand. Baby or satellite myofascial trigger points to consider include the supinator, brachioradialis, and triceps brachii.

Myofascial Trigger Point Comment
Wrist and hand pain are a common feature of these myofascial trigger points, with noted

stiffness in the morning and increased pain on bending the fingers. Difficulty sustaining a grip on handles or golf clubs is reported because of a noticeable increase in weakness of the associated muscles. Changes in sensations include tingling, pins and needles, and numbness. The pain is often mistaken for tendinitis.

Practitioner Guidelines
Patient positioning
Patient is supine, with the forearm pronated.

Needle type
Use 0.25 to 0.30 mm × 30 mm needle.

Needling directions
Using flat palpation, direct the needle toward the radius.

Precautions
Needling slowly and with care will ensure that you avoid the median nerve, located in the superior lateral forearm.

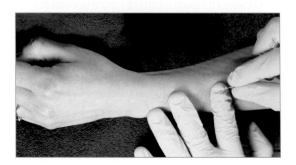

EXTENSOR CARPI RADIALIS LONGUS

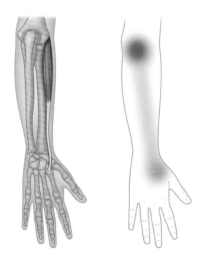

Latin, *extendere*, to extend; *carpi*, of the wrist; *radius*, staff, spoke of wheel; *longus*, long.

Origin
Lateral supracondylar ridge (inferior third) of the humerus, and lateral intermuscular septum.

Insertion
Dorsal base of the second metacarpal.

Nerve
Radial nerve C5–8.

Action
Extends and abducts the hand at the wrist joint.

Kinetic Chain Comment
Decelerates flexion of the wrist.

Myofascial Trigger Point Comment

Myofascial trigger points in this muscle lead to severe, unrelenting lateral epicondylitis (tennis elbow). Failure to treat these myofascial trigger points will result in the tennis elbow constantly returning—a great example of treating the symptom and not the cause. My patients complain of an unrelenting burning sensation with a focus on the elbow and referred pain into the wrist and the fleshy part between the thumb and the second digit, known as the "anatomical snuffbox."

Practitioner Guidelines

Patient positioning

Patient is supine, with the forearm pronated.

Needle type

Use 0.25 to 0.30 mm × 30 mm needle.

Needling directions

Using a pincer grip, direct the needle toward the radius.

Precautions

Needling slowly and with care will ensure that you avoid the median nerve, located in the superior lateral forearm.

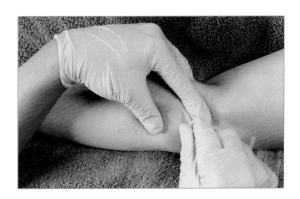

EXTENSOR DIGITORUM

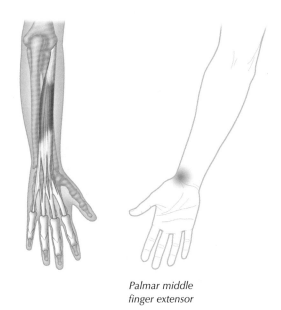

*Palmar middle
finger extensor*

Latin, *extendere*, to extend; *digitorum*, of the fingers/toes.

Origin

Lateral epicondyle of the humerus.

Insertion

Extensor expansions of the medial four digits.

Nerve

Posterior interosseous nerve C6–8.

Action

Extends the medial four digits (not the thumb) at the metacarpophalangeal joints. Extends the hand at the wrist joint.

Kinetic Chain Comment

Decelerator of the fingers, hands, and wrist through flexion. A good assessment is the finger flexion test, where the patient is asked to touch the pads of their fingers, i.e., fingertips, to the palmar pads while the metacarpophalangeal joints are held straight. All fingers should touch the palmar surface; failure to do so would demonstrate shortness in the muscle(s), most likely requiring treatment. Extensor digitorum is responsible for satellite myofascial trigger points in supinator, brachioradialis, extensor carpi radialis longus, and extensor carpi ulnaris.

Myofascial Trigger Point Comment
Pain, stiffness, cramping, and weakness are the common sensations reported, with pain traveling down the forearm to the posterior part of the hand into the middle finger. Pain can be confused with lateral epicondylitis, C7 radiculopathy, and de Quervain's stenosing tenosynovitis. All the associated muscles—such as the extensor indicis, digitorum, and digiti minimi—must be considered and appropriately treated when pain in the fingers is the chief complaint.

Practitioner Guidelines
Patient positioning
Patient is supine, with the forearm pronated or partially pronated.

Needle type
Use 0.25 to 0.30 mm × 30 mm needle.

Needling directions
Using a pincer grip, direct the needle toward the radius. This muscle is slightly medial and posterior to the brachioradialis muscle and can be targeted by moving the needle accordingly.

Precautions
Needling slowly and with care will ensure that you avoid the median nerve, located in the superior lateral forearm.

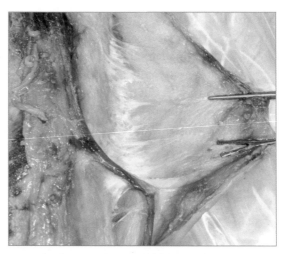

Here the forearm flexors reflect the close relationship of the forearm muscles. Note the ulnar nerve and artery on the medial aspect of the forearm. The deep fascia is clearly seen running in every direction. (Photograph: J. Sharkey 2010.)

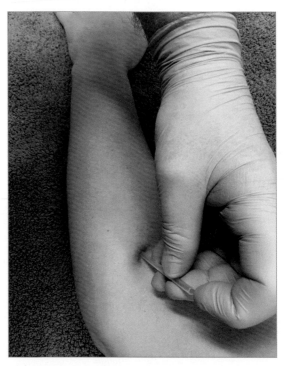

Flat or pincer palpation can be used.

FLEXOR CARPI ULNARIS

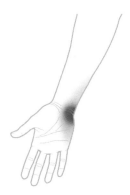

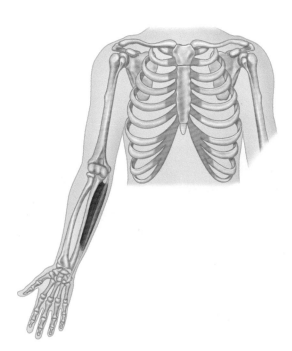

Latin, *flectere*, to bend; *carpi*, of the wrist; *ulnaris*, relating to the elbow/arm.

Origin
Humeral head: Medial epicondyle of the humerus.
Ulnar head: Olecranon process, and proximal posterior ulna.

Insertion
Base of the second metacarpal/pisiform bone, and a portion of the third metacarpal (hamate) and fifth metacarpal bones.

Nerve
Ulnar nerve C7, C8, T1.

Action
Both flexes and abducts the wrist and provides weak pronation of the forearm and elbow flexion.

Kinetic Chain Comment
Decelerates flexion and abduction of the wrist and hand and extension of the forearm at the elbow.

Myofascial Trigger Point Comment
Numbness and burning sensations can be experienced in the third to fifth digits. Pain is reported on the medial aspect (little-finger side) of the wrist as a sharp pain that can spread across the wrist joint, giving rise to a misdiagnosis of carpal tunnel or wrist sprains, medial epicondylitis, ulnar neuropathy, carpal tunnel syndrome, Charcot arthropathy, rheumatoid arthritis, osteoarthritis, C5 radiculopathy, peripheral neuropathy, Dupuytren's contracture, diabetic neuropathy, polyneuropathy, systemic lupus erythematosus, complex regional pain syndrome (reflex sympathetic dystrophy), and systemic infections or inflammation.

Of course, these must be ruled out by a primary medical practitioner, and so if in doubt, refer.

Practitioner Guidelines

Patient positioning
Patient is supine, with the forearm partially pronated.

Needle type
Use 0.25 to 0.30 mm × 30 mm needle.

Needling directions
The individual flexor muscles are identified and needled in a superior to inferior direction, using an angled motion.

Precautions
Needling slowly and with care will ensure that you avoid the radial nerve or posterior interosseous nerve. Insert the needle using a tangential approach to ensure you avoid placing the needle too deep into this compartment. The median nerve runs deep to this muscle. Excellent palpation skills are essential to ensure that the posterior interosseous nerve is located through flat palpation before needling.

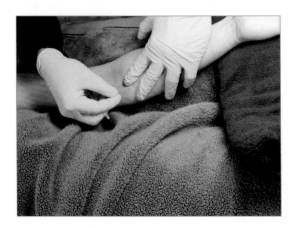

SUPINATOR

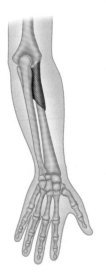

Latin, *supinus*, lying on the back.

Origin
Lateral epicondyle of the humerus, radial collateral ligament of the elbow joint, and annular ligament of the radius, including the superior crest of the ulna.

Insertion
Lateral upper one-third of the radius.

Nerve
Deep branch of radial nerve C5–7.

Action
Supinates the forearm and the hand.

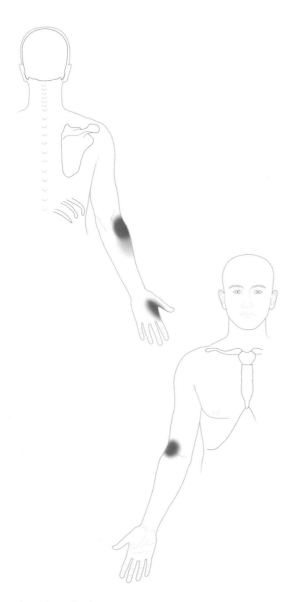

numbness and weakness in the hand (which may be due to compression of the deep branch of the radial nerve—the posterior interosseous nerve) and in the fingers.

Practitioner Guidelines

Patient positioning
Patient is supine, with the forearm supinated.

Needle type
Use 0.25 to 0.30 mm × 30 mm needle.

Needling directions
Insert the needle slowly, deep to brachioradialis while avoiding the cubital fossa, which will allow the patient to provide feedback. If the needle is close to the superficial sensory branch of the radial nerve, the patient will report discomfort early allowing the therapist to redirect the needle.

Precautions
Needling slowly and with care will ensure that you avoid the median nerve, which runs between the flexor digitorum superficialis and the flexor digitorum profundus. Working slowly allows time for the patient to give important feedback, and time for the therapist to take avoidance action.

Kinetic Chain Comment
Supinator is associated with deceleration of the elbow during extension. When the forearm is held between supination and pronation, the supinator will decelerate elbow extension.

Myofascial Trigger Point Comment
Supinator is a lateral elbow pain generator. The muscle sneaks pain down into the web of the thumb on the dorsal side. Changes in sensations include, but are not limited to,

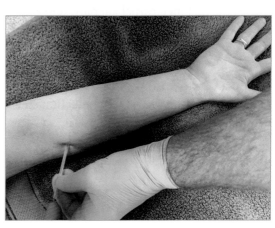

OPPONENS POLLICIS

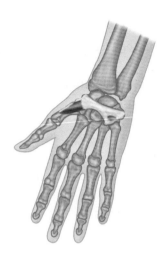

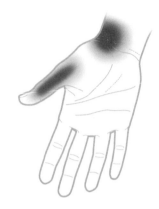

Latin, *opponens*, opposing; *pollicis*, of the thumb.

Origin
Flexor retinaculum, and tubercles of the scaphoid and trapezium.

Insertion
Lateral side of the first metacarpal.

Nerve
Median nerve C6–8, T1.

Action
Moves the first metacarpal laterally, opposing the thumb, toward the center of the palm and rotating it medially.

Kinetic Chain Comment
Opponens pollicis decelerates adduction and extension on the return from opposition. Problems with this muscle may lead to what Travell and Simons say patients refer to as a "clumsy thumb."

Myofascial Trigger Point Comment
Pain refers to the palmar surface of both the thumb and the wrist. It has been reported that many patients can identify a specific point on the radial side of the palmar aspect of the wrist as being the source of the pain.

Pain has been mistaken for C6 or C7 radiculopathy, carpal tunnel syndrome, de Quervain's stenosing tenosynovitis, carpometacarpal dysfunction, osteoarthritis, articular dysfunction, paronychia (ingrown thumbnail), bone cancer, bone fracture, strain/sprain, rheumatoid arthritis, Dupuytren's contracture, ganglion cyst, mixed connective tissue disease, Raynaud's phenomenon, frostbite, diabetic neuropathy, systemic infections or inflammation, nutritional inadequacy, metabolic imbalance, and toxicity and side effects of medications.

Practitioner Guidelines
Patient positioning
Patient is supine, with the forearm supported.

Needle type
Use 0.14 to 0.16 mm × 15 mm needle.

Needling directions
A fine/thin gauged needle is inserted along the anterior medial border of the first metacarpal aiming toward the thenar eminence.

Precautions
Fine, short needles are recommended.

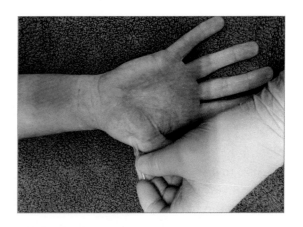

PALMARIS LONGUS

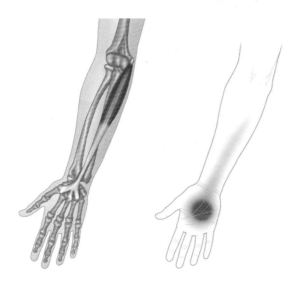

Latin, *palmaris*, relating to the palm; *longus*, long.

Palmaris longus is a meaty muscle with a substantial gaster and long tendon. It is interesting to note how the red muscle fibers run along the entire (or almost) length of this tendon (see image below). It is also worth noting the fascial slips attaching this muscle to neighboring fasciae and perimysial tissues.

Origin
Medial epicondyle of the humerus.

Insertion
Distal half of the flexor retinaculum, palmar aponeurosis, and transverse carpal ligament.

Nerve
Median nerve C7, C8, T1.

Action
Flexes the hand at the wrist, stiffens the aponeurosis of the palm, and assists in pronation and flexion of the forearm.

Kinetic Chain Comment
Decelerates extension of the hand at the wrist while decelerating supination of the hand against gravity and extension of the forearm at the elbow.

Myofascial Trigger Point Comment
A focal point of pain from the palmaris longus is experienced as a needle-like sensation, rather than the deep aching pain of myofascial trigger points in many other muscles. Pain can extend to the base of the thumb and the distal

crease of the palm. A residue of this pain can travel to the distal volar forearm.

Practitioner Guidelines

Patient positioning
Patient is supine, with the forearm supinated.

Needle type
Use 0.25 to 0.30 mm × 30 mm needle.

Needling directions
Using flat palpation, direct the needle at right angles to the skin, remembering that palmaris longus lies medial to flexor carpi radialis.

Precautions
Needling slowly and with care will ensure that you avoid going too deep. The median nerve courses between flexor digitorum superficialis and flexor digitorum profundus, and the ulnar nerve runs between flexor carpi ulnaris and flexor digitorum profundus (see page 146). Both should be avoided.

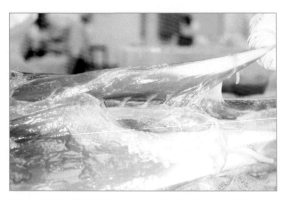

Palmaris longus (Photograph: J. Sharkey, 2010).

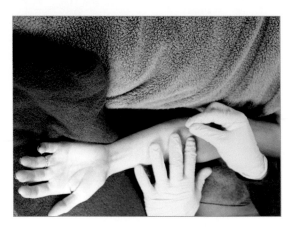

Muscles of the Hip and Thigh

GLUTEUS MAXIMUS

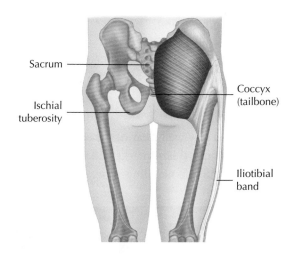

Sacrum

Ischial
tuberosity

Coccyx
(tailbone)

Iliotibial
band

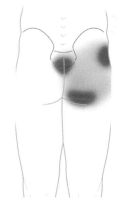

*Referral pattern of TrPs in the lower midportion of
the muscle, over the ischial tuberosity midpoint*

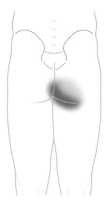

*Referral pattern of TrPs in the lower area of
the interior edge (medial inferior) of the muscle*

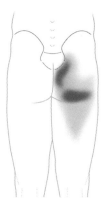

*Referral pattern of TrPs along the sacrum area
(superior medial) of the muscle*

Greek, *gloutos*, buttock. **Latin**, *maximus*, biggest.

Origin
Gluteal surface of the ilium behind the posterior gluteal line, posterior border of the ilium, aponeurosis of the erector spinae, sacrotuberous ligament, and gluteal aponeurosis.

Insertion
Iliotibial tract of the fascia lata, and gluteal tuberosity of the femur by means of a broad aponeurosis.

Nerve
Inferior gluteal nerve L5, S1, S2.

Action
Laterally rotates and extends the hip joint and assists in adduction at the hip joint. Eccentrically, the gluteus maximus contracts to decelerate hip flexion, adduction, and internal rotation.

Kinetic Chain Comment
Gluteus maximus plays a significant role in stabilizing both the sacroiliac joint and the knee joint. It does so by means of superior fibers, which attach to the aponeurosis of the sacrotuberous ligament, and inferior fibers, which attach anteriorly to the iliotibial tract, providing tension down to the knee. Weak gluteal muscles have wide-reaching implications up and down the kinetic chain.

Myofascial Trigger Point Comment
It is hypothesized that gluteal myofascial trigger points could be a result of inhibition in the gluteal muscles caused by spasm in the psoas muscles, gluteus medius, and gluteus minimus. The formation of these myofascial trigger points provides much-needed tension for sacroiliac support. Pain is often felt in the lower back and mimics bursitis of the hip, with pain experienced at the site of the coccygeal bone and of the gluteal crease.

Practitioner Guidelines
Patient positioning
Patient is side lying, with the anatomical leg supported by an appropriate bolster.

Needle type
Use 0.25 to 0.30 mm × 30 mm needle.

Needling directions
Therapist depresses the skin and subcutis to the depth of the muscle fibers. Flat palpation is recommended.

Precautions
Take care to stay well clear of the sciatic nerve. Check anatomical landmarks and ensure that you are in the safe needling zone.

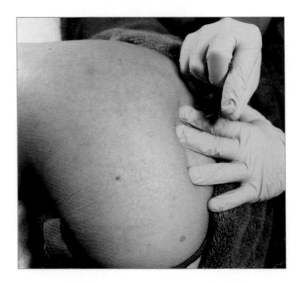

GLUTEUS MEDIUS

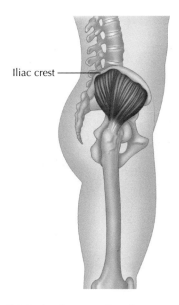

Iliac crest

TrPs in the gluteus medius often occur in a line along and below the iliac crest

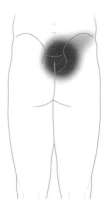

Referral pattern of TrPs usually found under the front portion of the muscle along and under the iliac crest

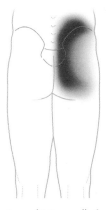

Referral pattern of TrPs usually found under the back portion of the muscle close to the sacrum, along and under the iliac crest

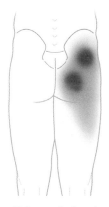

Referral pattern of TrPs usually found under the middle portion of the muscle along and under the iliac crest

Greek, *gloutos*, buttock. **Latin**, *medius*, middle.

Origin
Outer surface of the ilium, between the posterior and middle gluteal lines.

Insertion
Posterolateral surface of the greater trochanter of the femur.

Nerve
Superior gluteal nerve L4, L5, S1.

Action
Abducts and both externally/internally rotates the hip. Tilts the pelvis when walking.

Kinetic Chain Comment

Gluteus medius is a crucial muscle in offering stability to the lateral line. Weakness leads to lower back pain for runners and creates undue knee stress, which is often mistaken for discogenic problems and sacroiliac dysfunction. The one-leg standing test (Stork test) will often result in the patient being unable to stabilize the iliofemoral relationship on the frontal plane, because gluteus medius is required to eccentrically contract or decelerate the movement. This can be evident as an exaggerated lateral hip-sway during walking, which results from over-pronation of the foot, dropped arch, rotation of the second toe (Morton's foot), and medial rotation of the tibia/femur.

Baby or satellite myofascial trigger points include the quadratus lumborum, piriformis, gluteus minimus, gluteus maximus, and tensor fasciae latae.

Myofascial Trigger Point Comment

Lower back pain is felt above and below the belt line. Pain in the hips makes it difficult to sleep in comfort and leads to disturbed sleep patterns. This muscle is a major generator of lower back and hip pain, as well as being responsible for complaints of a burning sensation along the posterior superior iliac spine (PSIS) and sacroiliac joint. Pain is often mistaken for lumbago-type pain, with discomfort (such as tenderness) into the buttocks and superior thigh.

Practitioner Guidelines

Patient positioning

Patient is side lying on the unaffected side, with the leg to be treated suitably supported.

Needle type

Use 0.25 to 0.30 mm × 30 mm needle.

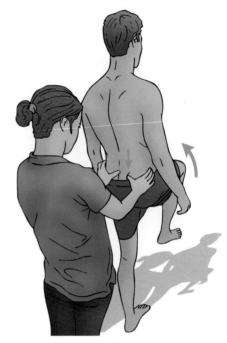

Stork test.

Needling directions

Therapist depresses the skin and subcutis to the depth of the muscle fibers. Flat palpation is recommended.

Precautions

Take care to stay well clear of the sciatic nerve. Check anatomical landmarks and ensure that you are in the safe needling zone. Needle the gaster of the muscle to avoid associated neurovascular structures.

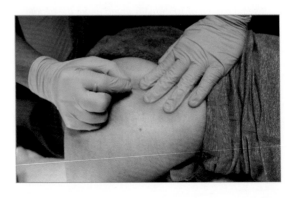

GLUTEUS MINIMUS

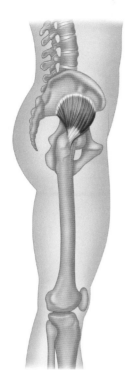

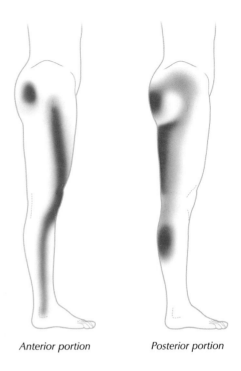

Anterior portion   *Posterior portion*

Greek, *gloutos*, buttock. **Latin**, *minimus*, smallest.

Origin
Outer surface of the ilium, between the middle and inferior gluteal lines.

Insertion
Anterior surface of the greater trochanter of the femur.

Nerve
Superior gluteal nerve L4, L5, S1.

Action
Abducts and medially rotates the hip. Assists in tilting the pelvis when walking.

Kinetic Chain Comment
Acts to decelerate external rotation and adduction of the femur in the hip joint.

Myofascial Trigger Point Comment
Pain is experienced in the posterior and/or lateral thigh as well as deep in the buttocks. Numbness can be another symptom, and pain can refer as far as the lateral ankle. Such pain and discomfort can be mistaken for sciatic pain.

Practitioner Guidelines
Patient positioning
Patient is side lying on the unaffected side, with a supporting bolster under the leg to be treated.

Needle type
Use 0.25 to 0.30 mm × 30 mm needle.

Needling directions

Therapist depresses the skin and subcutis to the depth of the muscle fibers. Flat palpation is recommended.

Precautions

Take care to stay well clear of the sciatic nerve. Check anatomical landmarks and ensure that you are in the safe needling zone.

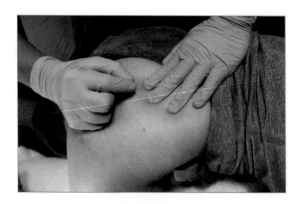

TENSOR FASCIAE LATAE

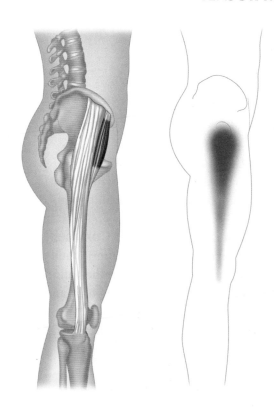

Latin, *tendere*, to stretch, pull; *fasciae*, band; *latae*, side or lateral.

Origin

Anterior superior iliac spine, outer lip of the anterior iliac crest, and fascia lata.

Insertion

Iliotibial tract.

Nerve

Superior gluteal nerve L4, L5, S1.

Action

Assists in stabilizing and steadying the hip and knee joints by putting tension on the iliotibial tract of fascia.

Kinetic Chain Comment

Tensor fasciae latae is a vitally important structure in providing stability through the knee and pelvis. This muscle is a junction for several chains, including the spiral and lateral chains. The anteromedial fibers are responsible for flexion of the thigh, while the posterolateral fibers provide stability to the knee. Tensor fasciae latae assists various muscles, including the gluteus medius and minimus, rectus femoris, iliopsoas, pectineus, and sartorius.

Myofascial Trigger Point Comment

Pain is felt at the level of the greater trochanter in the hip joint. Walking and running activities make the pain more intense. Pain can refer midway down the lateral thigh and can cause additional knee pain.

Practitioner Guidelines
Patient positioning
Patient can be supine, or side lying on the unaffected side with the leg to be treated suitably supported.

Needle type
Use 0.25 to 0.30 mm × 30 mm needle.

Needling directions
The muscle is identified and needled in a superior to inferior direction.

Precautions
Needle toward the femur.

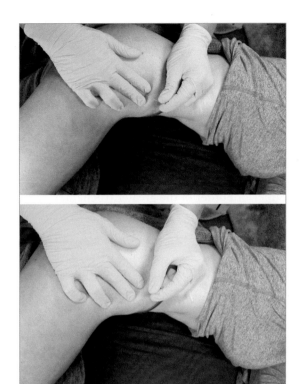

Side lying with the leg supported.

PIRIFORMIS

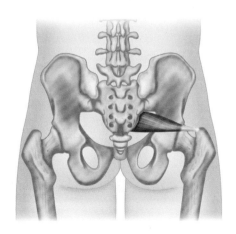

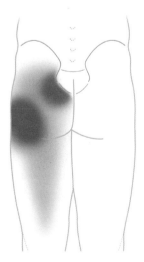

Latin, *pirum*, pear; *forma*, shape.

Origin
Second to fourth costotransverse joints of the anterior sacrum. Small number of fibers arise from the superior border of the greater sciatic notch.

Insertion
Superior border of the greater trochanter of the femur.

Nerve
Ventral rami of lumbar nerve L5, and sacral nerves S1, S2.

Action
Laterally rotates the hip and abducts the thigh when the hip is flexed.

Kinetic Chain Comment
Piriformis eccentrically contracts to decelerate internal rotation and hip adduction when the hip is flexed. A short piriformis can cause the sacrum to tilt, giving the appearance of a short-leg discrepancy, and result in a rotation or twisting of the sacrum in the sacroiliac joint, setting up additional sacroiliac stress. If not corrected in a timely fashion, this is a recipe for shoulder injury.

Myofascial Trigger Point Comment
Pain is felt in the buttock, hip, and base of the spine, including the sacral base and at times into the upper hamstrings.

Practitioner Guidelines
Patient positioning
Patient is prone.

Needle type
Use 0.25 to 0.30 mm × 30 mm needle.

Needling directions
Piriformis is located lateral to the greater sciatic foramen, and the needle should be directed in a medial to lateral direction, bearing in mind the underlying nerve structure. Work slowly and look for patient feedback. This application can also be used for the associated gemelli muscles.

Precautions
The sciatic nerve, which runs under the piriformis (and in some cases over or through the muscle), must be avoided.

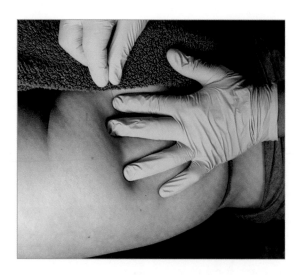

GEMELLI

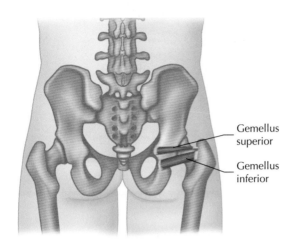

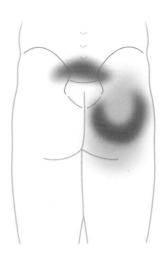

Gemellus superior
Gemellus inferior

Latin, *gemellus*, twin/double.

Origin
Inferior: Upper border of the ischial tuberosity.
Superior: Spine of the ischium.

Insertion
Middle part of the medial aspect of the greater trochanter of the femur (inferior and superior).

Nerve
Nerve to quadratus femoris L4, L5, S1 (inferior). Nerve to obturator internus L5, S1, S2 (superior).

Action
Laterally rotates and stabilizes the hip.

Kinetic Chain Comment
Any pain in the pelvic area will result in either an apprehension of movement or a reluctance to move. This often results in postural adaptations and changes in muscle synergies to carry out some function.

Myofascial Trigger Point Comment
Intrapelvic pain is felt, with difficulty sitting for even short periods of time. Intense and unrelenting pain can be referred into the base of the spine and into the gluteal area. The gemelli are difficult to treat with finger applications but myofascial trigger points can be treated successfully with dry needling.

Practitioner Guidelines
Patient positioning
Patient is prone.

Needle type
Use 0.25 to 0.30 mm × 30 mm needle.

Needling directions

Gemelli are located lateral to the greater sciatic foramen, and the needle should be directed in a medial to lateral direction, bearing in mind the underlying nerve structure. Work slowly and look for patient feedback.

Precautions

The sciatic nerve must be avoided.

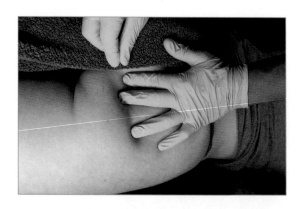

OBTURATOR INTERNUS

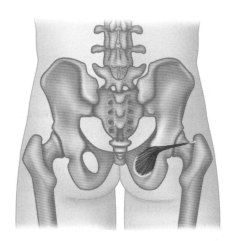

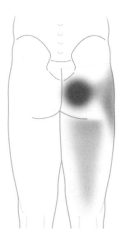

Latin, *obturare*, to obstruct; *internus*, internal.

Origin

Pelvic surface of the obturator membrane, and bony margin of the obturator foramen.

Insertion

Anterior part of the medial surface of the greater trochanter of the femur.

Nerve

Branch of ventral rami of lumbar nerve L5, and sacral nerves S1, S2.

Action

Laterally rotates the extended thigh at the hip, stabilizes the hip, and produces horizontal extension. Abducts the flexed thigh.

Kinetic Chain Comment

Eccentric contraction of obturator internus decelerates internal rotation of the femur, while pulling the head of the femur into the acetabulum to fix the femoral head during abduction. It eccentrically controls the head of the femur on returning from adduction.

Myofascial Trigger Point Comment

Local pain is experienced deep within the pelvic basin and out as far as the anterior medial portion of the greater trochanter.

Practitioner Guidelines

Patient positioning
Patient is prone.

Needle type
Use 0.25 to 0.30 mm × 30 mm needle.

Needling directions
Obturator internus is located lateral to the greater sciatic foramen, and the needle should be directed in a medial to lateral direction, bearing in mind the underlying nerve structure. Work slowly and look for patient feedback.

Precautions
The sciatic nerve must be avoided.

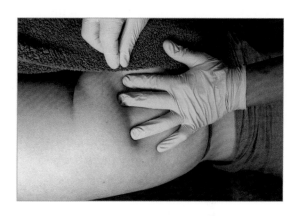

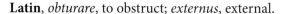

OBTURATOR EXTERNUS

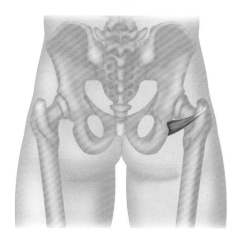

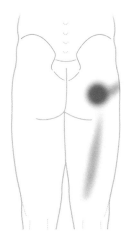

Latin, *obturare*, to obstruct; *externus*, external.

Origin
Rami of the pubis, and ischium.

Insertion
Trochanteric fossa of the femur.

Nerve
Posterior division of obturator nerve L3, L4.

Action
Laterally rotates and stabilizes the hip.

Kinetic Chain Comment

Eccentric contraction of obturator externus decelerates medial or internal rotation and abduction of the femur.

Myofascial Trigger Point Comment

Local pain is experienced deep within the pelvic basin and out as far as the posterior portion of the greater trochanter. If resisted, medial rotation causes an increase in pain (sometimes the pain shoots down the medial aspect of the femur). I have found that myofascial trigger points housed in the obturator externus may well be the culprit. Resisted medial rotation may therefore be a worthwhile test to perform.

Practitioner Guidelines

Patient positioning

Patient is prone.

Needle type

Use 0.25 to 0.30 mm × 30 mm needle.

Needling directions

Obturator externus is located lateral to the greater sciatic foramen, and the needle should be directed in a medial to lateral direction, bearing in mind the underlying nerve structure. Work slowly and look for patient feedback.

Precautions

The sciatic nerve must be avoided.

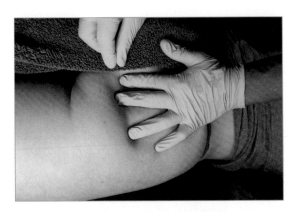

QUADRATUS FEMORIS

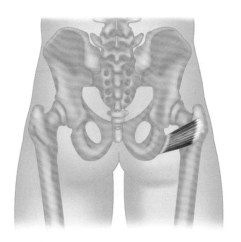
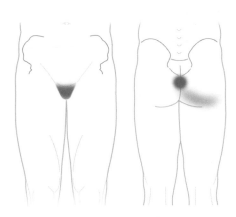

Latin, *quadratus*, squared; *femoris*, of the thigh.

Origin
Lateral border (superior aspect) of the ischial tuberosity.

Insertion
Quadrate tubercle of the femur, and a vertical line below this to the level of the lesser trochanter.

Nerve
Nerve to quadratus femoris L4, L5, S1.

Action
Laterally rotates and stabilizes the hip.

Kinetic Chain Comment
Quadratus femoris eccentrically decelerates medial rotation of the femur at the hip.

Myofascial Trigger Point Comment
Pain is felt locally in the posterior pubis and lower gluteal area. Difficulty sleeping and walking downstairs are reported.

Practitioner Guidelines
Patient positioning
Patient is prone.

Needle type
Use 0.25 to 0.30 mm × 30 mm needle.

Needling directions
Muscle is identified and needled with a straight in-and-out motion.

Precautions
Avoid the sciatic nerve, which runs almost midline and is palpable at a thumb width just beneath the gluteal crease.

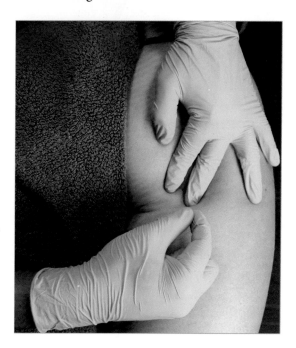

ADDUCTOR LONGUS

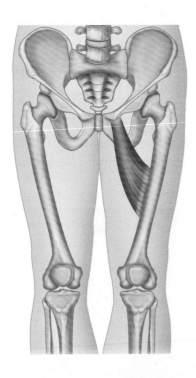

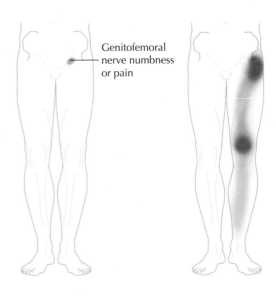

Genitofemoral nerve numbness or pain

Latin, *adducere*, to lead to; *longus*, long.

Origin
Anterior of the pubis in an angle between the crest and the symphysis.

Insertion
Middle third of the medial lip of the linea aspera.

Nerve
Anterior division of obturator nerve L2–L4.

Action
Adducts the hip joint. Flexes the extended femur at the hip joint. Extends the flexed femur at the hip joint. Assists in lateral rotation of the hip joint.

Kinetic Chain Comment
Adductor longus decelerates femoral external rotation and abduction of the thigh.

Myofascial Trigger Point Comment
Myofascial trigger points in adductor longus should be considered when patients present with groin pain. Pain can be felt deep in the hip joint, in the inner thigh, and at the medial aspect of the knee. Sensations such as joint stiffness in the hip are reported, restricting the range of motion in all directions.

Practitioner Guidelines
Patient positioning
Patient is supine, with the hip and knee of the leg to be treated in flexion and the hip externally rotated. Alternatively, the patient can be side lying and positioned on the involved limb, with that hip and knee extended while the other leg is flexed at the hip and knee (moving it out of the way) and is suitably supported.

Needle type
Use 0.25 to 0.30 mm × 30 to 50 mm needle.

Needling directions
Using pincer palpation, locate and secure the myofascial trigger point within the palpable taut band. Insert the needle and direct it toward your finger.

Precautions
Avoid needling the femoral nerve, artery, and vein, as well as the obturator nerve.

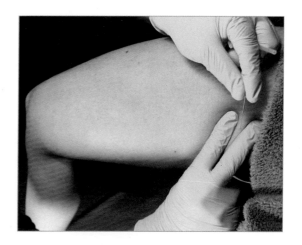

ADDUCTOR MAGNUS

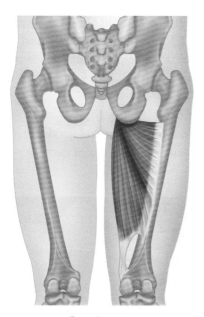

Posterior view

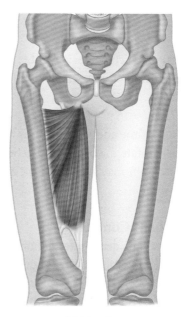

Anterior view

Latin, *adducere*, to lead to; *magnus*, large.

Origin
Anterior fibers: Inferior or anterior ramus of the pubis, in the angle between the crest and the symphysis.
Posterior fibers: Ischial tuberosity.

Insertion
Entire length of the femur, extending from the gluteal tuberosity along the linea aspera, medial supracondylar line, and adductor tubercle on the medial condyle of the femur.

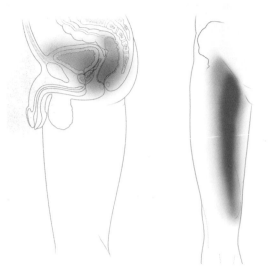

Pelvic referral pattern for TrPs in the high adductor magnus

Nerve

Tibial portion of sciatic nerve L4, L5, S1.
Posterior division of obturator nerve L2–4.

Action

Upper fibers of the adductor magnus adduct and laterally rotate the hip joint. Vertical fibers from the ischium may assist in weak extension of the hip joint.

Kinetic Chain Comment

Adductor magnus decelerates femoral external rotation and abduction of the thigh.

Myofascial Trigger Point Comment

Pain referred from adductor magnus can manifest itself in many ways, including deep pelvic pain, and pubic, bladder, rectal, or vaginal pain. This pain can often be mistaken for serious visceral or gynecological pathology. When pathology is not clear, myofascial trigger points should be investigated as the root cause of this severe pain.

Practitioner Guidelines

Patient positioning

Patient is supine, with the hip and knee of the leg to be treated in flexion and the hip externally rotated.

Needle type

Use 0.25 to 0.30 mm × 30 to 50 mm needle.

Needling directions

Using pincer palpation, locate and secure the myofascial trigger point within the palpable taut band. Insert the needle and direct it toward your fingers, in an anterior to posterior direction.

Precautions

Avoid needling the femoral nerve, artery, and vein, as well as the obturator nerve.

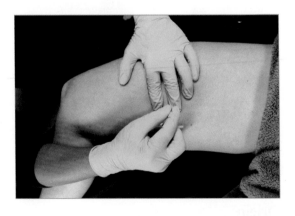

ADDUCTOR BREVIS

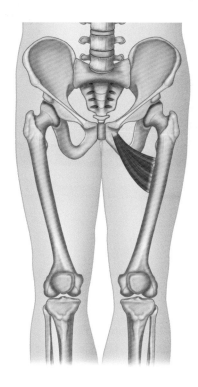

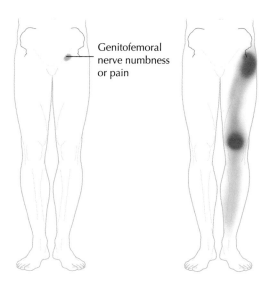

Genitofemoral nerve numbness or pain

Latin, *adducere*, to lead to; *brevis*, short.

Origin
Outer surface of the inferior ramus of the pubis.

Insertion
On a line extending from the lesser trochanter to the upper part of the linea aspera.

Nerve
Anterior division of obturator nerve L2–4.

Action
Adducts the hip joint. Flexes the extended femur at the hip joint. Extends the flexed femur at the hip joint. Assists in lateral rotation of the hip joint.

Kinetic Chain Comment
Adductor brevis decelerates femoral external rotation and abduction of the thigh.

Myofascial Trigger Point Comment
Pain is felt deep in the hip, predominantly on the medial side of the thigh and referring to the medial aspect of the knee joint, which can be mistaken for arthritic pain.

Practitioner Guidelines
Patient positioning
Patient is supine, with the hip and knee of the leg to be treated in flexion and the hip externally rotated. Alternatively, the patient can be side lying and positioned on the involved limb, with that hip and knee extended while the other leg is flexed at the hip and knee (moving it out of the way) and is suitably supported.

Needle type
Use 0.25 to 0.30 mm × 30 to 50 mm needle.

Needling directions

Using pincer palpation, locate and secure the myofascial trigger point within the palpable taut band. Insert the needle and direct it toward your finger.

Precautions

Avoid needling the femoral nerve, artery, and vein, as well as the obturator nerve.

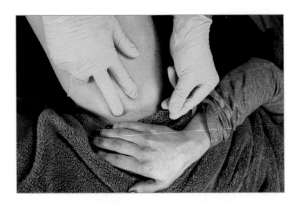

GRACILIS

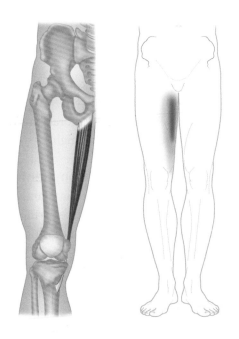

Latin, *gracilis*, slender, delicate.

Origin

Anterior lower half of the symphysis pubis, and medial margin of the inferior ramus of the pubis.

Insertion

Front and medial surface of the shaft of the tibia, just below the condyle.

Nerve

Anterior division of obturator nerve L2–4.

Action

Adducts the hip joint. Flexes the knee joint. Medially rotates the knee joint when flexed.

Kinetic Chain Comment

Gracilis decelerates femoral external rotation and abduction of the thigh.

Myofascial Trigger Point Comment

Myofascial trigger points can not only refer pain but also produce changes in sensation; gracilis is a good example of that. Patients complain of a hot and stinging feeling on the inner thigh, just superficial to the skin.

Practitioner Guidelines

Patient positioning

Patient is supine, with the hip and knee of the leg to be treated in flexion and the hip externally rotated.

Needle type

Use 0.25 to 0.30 mm × 30 to 50 mm needle.

Needling directions

Gracilis lies posterior to the adductor longus. Using pincer palpation, locate and secure the myofascial trigger point within the palpable taut band. Insert the needle perpendicular to the skin and direct it using a shallow angle. Using the correct depth (muscle gaster only) will ensure that no neurovascular tissues will be encountered.

Precautions

Avoid needling the femoral nerve, artery, and vein, as well as the obturator nerve.

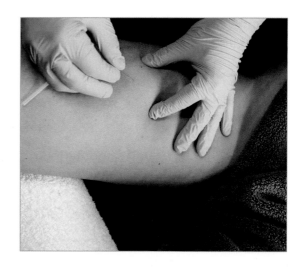

PECTINEUS

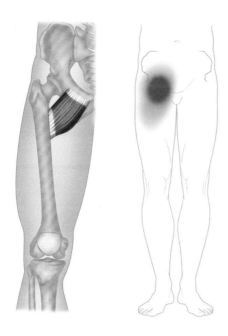

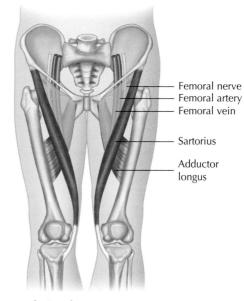

Femoral triangle.

Latin, *pecten*, comb; *pectinatus*, comb shaped.

Origin

Pectineal line of the pubis, between the iliopubic eminence and the pubic tubercle.

Insertion

Pectineal line of the femur, from the lesser trochanter to the linea aspera.

Nerve

Femoral and obturator nerves L2–4.

Action
Adducts the hip joint. Flexes the hip joint.

Kinetic Chain Comment
Pectineus decelerates femoral external rotation and abduction of the thigh.

Myofascial Trigger Point Comment
Pain is felt deeply in the groin as a sharp pain within the femoral triangle. Similar to the adductor muscle group, the pain is sometimes felt in the joint itself.

Practitioner Guidelines
Patient positioning
Patient is supine, with the hip slightly externally rotated.

Needle type
Use 0.25 to 0.30 mm × 30 to 50 mm needle.

Needling directions
Before needling, locate the femoral artery and maintain a finger on top of it. Using flat palpation, identify the myofascial trigger point within the palpable taut band just medial to the femoral artery. Insert the needle and direct it into the myofascial trigger, toward the muscle.

Precautions
Avoid needling the femoral nerve, artery, and vein, as well as the obturator nerve.

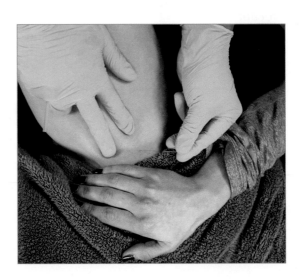

HAMSTRINGS

German, *hamme*, back of leg. **Latin**, *stringere*, to draw together.

Origin
Hamstrings arise from the ischial tuberosity. Biceps femoris blends a long head with the sacrotuberous ligament, and its short head attaches in the linea aspera and intermuscular septum.

Insertion
Semitendinosus and semimembranosus attach to the posteromedial tibia by means of the tibial condyle (semimembranosus) and the medial surface of the tibia, including the deep fascia (semitendinosus). Biceps femoris inserts on the lateral aspect of the fibula head and the lateral condyle of the tibia.

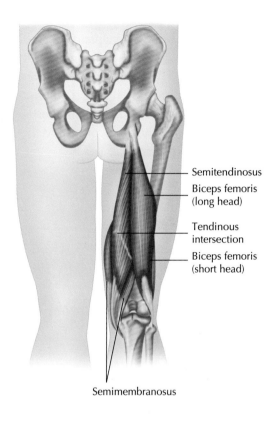

Semitendinosus

Biceps femoris
(long head)

Tendinous
intersection

Biceps femoris
(short head)

Semimembranosus

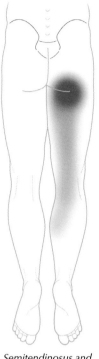

Semitendinosus and
semimembranosus

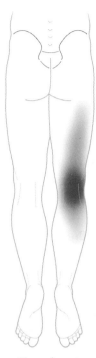

Biceps femoris

Nerve
Sciatic nerve L4, L5, S1–3.

Action
Hamstrings flex the knee joint. Semimembranosus and semitendinosus only medially rotate the knee joint, and assist in medial rotation of the hip joint when the knee is flexed. Biceps femoris laterally rotates the knee joint and assists in lateral rotation of the hip joint when the knee is flexed.

Kinetic Chain Comment
Hamstrings eccentrically contract during gait to decelerate extension of the knee joint and hip flexion, while also playing a very important role in pelvic stability and decelerate internal rotation on heel-strike. They disappear under gluteus maximus and provide force closure of the sacroiliac joint through the coupled action of the force provided by the contralateral latissimus dorsi. This force is transmitted through the sacrotuberous ligament and further up to the thoracolumbar fascia.

Myofascial Trigger Point Comment
Typically, pain is referred up toward the gluteal muscles, with some residual pain spreading down just below and behind the knee into the medial gaster of the gastrocnemius. This pain can often be mistaken for sciatic pain. Weak

inhibited gluteal muscles, including gluteus medius, can lead to myofascial trigger points forming in the hamstrings and lumbar erector muscles, including the quadratus lumborum. Ultimately, the hamstrings are trying to be gluteal muscles, while the lumbar muscles are trying to be hamstrings.

Practitioner Guidelines
Patient positioning
Patient is prone.

Needle type
Use 0.25 to 0.30 mm × 30 to 50 mm needle.

Needling directions
Using either flat or pincer palpation, locate and secure the myofascial trigger point within the palpable taut band. Insert the needle and direct it into the myofascial trigger point, toward the medial side (semimembranosus, semitendinosus) of the thigh, or toward the lateral side (biceps femoris).

Precautions
Avoid needling the sciatic nerve, which is located along the posterior midline of the thigh.

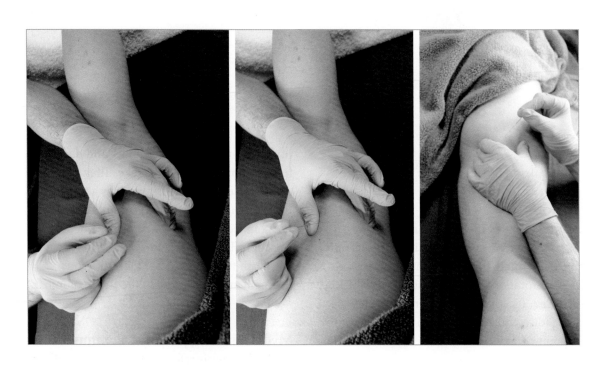

SARTORIUS

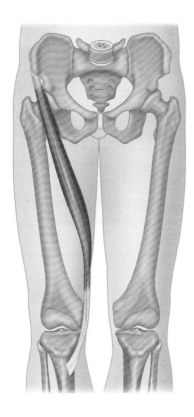

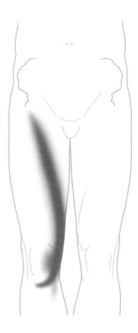

Latin, *sartor*, tailor.

Origin
Anterior superior iliac spine (ASIS).

Insertion
Superior aspect of the medial surface of the tibial shaft, near the tibial tuberosity.

Nerve
Anterior branch of femoral nerve L2–4.

Action
Flexes and laterally rotates the hip joint and flexes the knee (tailor's muscle).

Kinetic Chain Comment
Decelerates extension and medial rotation at the hip joint and extension at the knee. Muscles with baby or satellite myofascial trigger points to consider include rectus femoris, vastus medialis, pectineus, and the adductors.

Myofascial Trigger Point Comment
A severe burning or sharp tingling pain or sensation is experienced along the anterior but mostly medial aspect of the thigh and kneecap. Typically, this is not felt as a deep knee pain. Be sure to test for chondromalacia patellae (runner's knee).

Practitioner Guidelines
Patient positioning
Patient is supine, with the thigh slightly externally rotated.

Needle type
Use 0.25 to 0.30 mm × 30 mm needle.

Needling directions
Muscle is identified and needled using slightly angled in-and-out motions.

Precautions
The femoral neurovascular structures lie on the medial border of the sartorius, in the superior portion, while the muscle crosses over the neurovascular bundle from around midway down the femur. These nerves and blood vessels must be avoided.

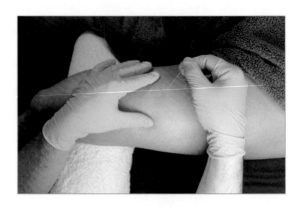

QUADRICEPS

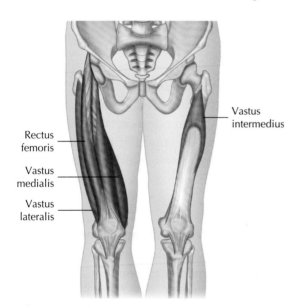

Rectus femoris

Vastus medialis

Vastus lateralis

Vastus intermedius

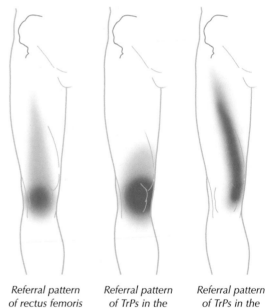

Referral pattern of rectus femoris

Referral pattern of TrPs in the lower muscle

Referral pattern of TrPs in the upper muscle

Latin, *quadriceps*, four-headed.

Some anatomists consider the vastus medialis obliquus fibers to be a separate and functionally distinct structure. These oblique fibers attach to the tendon of the rectus femoris and the medial border of the patella, and to the anterior medial condyle of the tibia.

It is interesting to note that the expansions which pass across the knee joint to attach to the tibia replace the joint capsule in this region, and then fuse with the deep fascia embracing the tibial tuberosity.

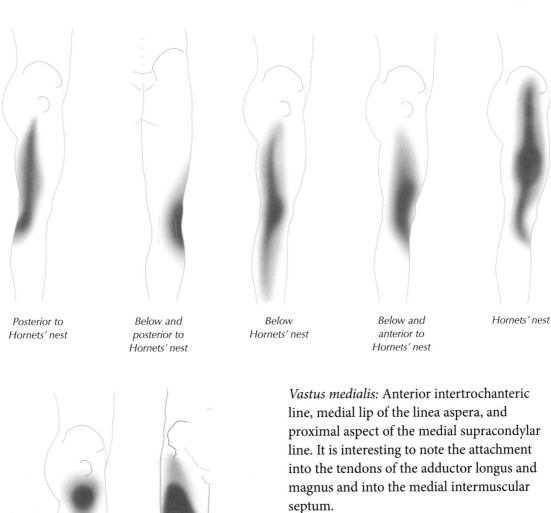

Posterior to
Hornets' nest

Below and
posterior to
Hornets' nest

Below
Hornets' nest

Below and
anterior to
Hornets' nest

Hornets' nest

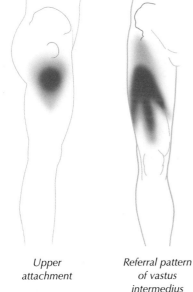

Upper
attachment

Referral pattern
of vastus
intermedius

Vastus medialis: Anterior intertrochanteric line, medial lip of the linea aspera, and proximal aspect of the medial supracondylar line. It is interesting to note the attachment into the tendons of the adductor longus and magnus and into the medial intermuscular septum.

Vastus lateralis: Intertrochanteric line and greater trochanter, gluteal tuberosity and lateral lip of the linea aspera, and lateral intermuscular septum.

Vastus intermedius: Anterior lateral surface of the proximal two-thirds of the femur, distal half of the linea aspera, and lateral intermuscular septum.

Articularis genu: Two slips from the anterior femur below the vastus intermedius (pulls the capsule superiorly).

Origin

Rectus femoris: Anterior inferior iliac spine (AIIS), and groove above the rim of the acetabulum.

Insertion

All the quadriceps wrap up the patella (sesamoid bone), with each having a unique and specific line of pull or directional force acting on the patella. They share a common tendon (patellar tendon or ligament) and attach to the tibial tuberosity.

Nerve

Femoral nerve L2–4.

Action

Extend the knee joint. Rectus femoris additionally flexes the hip joint.

Kinetic Chain Comment

Quadriceps have a significant impact on pelvic rotation (anterior), kneecap tracking, and knee positioning, and shortness of them can ultimately influence head and neck positioning, cause knee pain, and affect foot and ankle movement. Eccentric contraction decelerates knee flexion, adduction, and internal rotation during heel-strike of the gait cycle. Rectus femoris eccentrically decelerates hip extension and knee flexion during gait. The interrelationship of all the quadriceps muscles provides dynamic stability to the knee.

Myofascial Trigger Point Comment

Pain involves a deep toothache-like pain (vastus medialis) in the knee joint, or on the lateral or medial aspect of the thigh, including the knee.

Practitioner Guidelines

Patient positioning

Patient is supine, with a bolster placed under the knee for support.

Needle type

Use 0.25 to 0.30 mm × 30 mm needle.

Needling directions

Using flat palpation, locate and secure the myofascial trigger point within the palpable taut band. Insert the needle and direct it toward the anterior surface of the femur.

Precautions

Do not insert the whole length of the needle to avoid the branch of the femoral artery, which lies under the muscle.

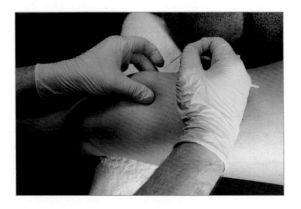

Muscles of the Leg and Foot

GASTROCNEMIUS

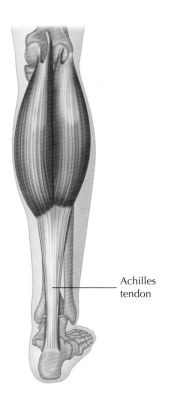

Achilles tendon

Greek, *gaster*, belly; *kneme*, lower leg.

Origin
Medial and lateral condyles of the femur (posteriorly), capsule of the knee joint, and oblique popliteal ligament.

Insertion
Posterior surface of calcaneus.

Nerve
Tibial nerve S1, S2.

Action
When we run or walk, gastrocnemius provides considerable forces, enough to propel our bodies in jumping. A powerful plantar flexor, the muscle contracts eccentrically to assist in decelerating femoral internal rotation and assists in external rotation of the knee during the push-off phase of gait and aids knee flexion during the swing phase.

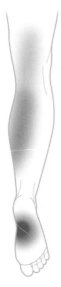

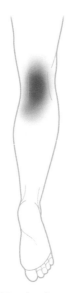

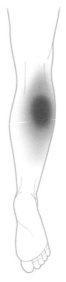

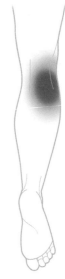

This referral pattern is from TrPs in the area of the upper medial head

This referral pattern is from TrPs in the extreme upper medial head and its tendon attachment

This referral pattern is from TrPs in the area of the middle lateral head

This referral pattern is from TrPs in the area of the upper medial head and its tendon attachment

Kinetic Chain Comment

The relationship with the heads of gastrocnemius and tendons of the hamstrings must be considered when participating in machine-based exercise. A shared fascia with the plantar muscles of the foot can highlight the need for balance, both up and down the kinetic chain. Eccentrically, the muscle decelerates ankle extension in gait.

Myofascial Trigger Point Comment

Several myofascial trigger points can form in this muscle, referring pain and a sense of stiffness or tension into the medial plantar aspect of the foot, and diffuse pain spread over one or both of the gasters. Pain can also refer up into the medial hamstrings. Typically, individuals will try to statically stretch the symptoms away; this will irritate the muscle spindle response and serve only to compound the symptoms. The posterior kinetic chain should be assessed to identify short hypertonic muscles and myofascial migration.

Practitioner Guidelines

Patient positioning
Patient is prone, with the ankles supported.

Needle type
Use 0.25 to 0.30 mm × 30 mm needle.

Needling directions
Identify the myofascial trigger point and insert the needle in either gaster, in a lateral to medial direction (medial head) or in a medial to lateral direction (lateral head), as shown in the image.

Precautions
Staying below the knee to avoid popliteal structures, the therapist must be aware of the location of the fibular, tibial, and sural nerves and associated vessels. Because of the proximity of the neurovascular structures, it is advised to work slowly and seek patient feedback.

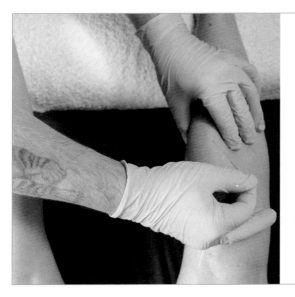
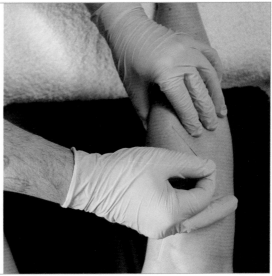

TIBIALIS ANTERIOR

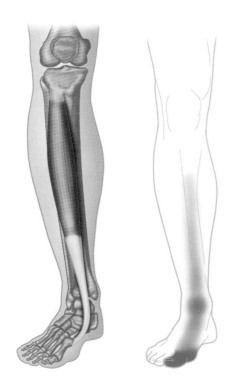

Latin, *tibialis*, relating to the shin; *anterior*, at the front.

Origin
Lateral condyle and proximal two-thirds of the lateral surface of the tibia, interosseous membrane, deep fascia, and lateral intermuscular septum.

Insertion
Medial and plantar surface of the medial cuneiform bone, and base of the metatarsal bone.

Nerve
Deep fibular nerve L4, L5, S1.

Action
Dorsiflexes the ankle joint and assists in inverting the foot. When contracting eccentrically, decelerates plantar flexion at heel-strike and eversion of the mid-foot in

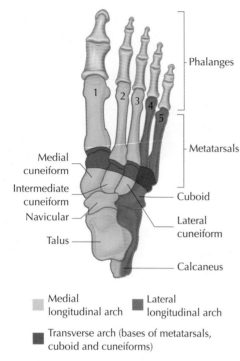

Foot arches.

mid-stance. Offers dynamic stabilization to the mid-tarsal joint and accelerates supination of the foot before heel-strike.

Kinetic Chain Comment

As a result of reciprocal inhibition, tibialis anterior can become weak, long, and tight, predisposing the foot to over-pronation and eversion (flat foot). Short, spastic, or contractured fibulares will facilitate this inhibition, thereby reducing soft tissue support to all three foot arches.

Myofascial Trigger Point Comment

Myofascial trigger points in tibialis anterior refer down into the great toe. Pain can also be experienced in the ankle (anteromedially) as the muscle tendon passes the retinaculum. Fallen arches in the foot place eccentric loads on tibialis anterior, while hypercontracted fibulares will increase inhibition in this

muscle—all in all, a recipe for myofascial trigger point evolution.

Practitioner Guidelines
Patient positioning
Patient is supine, with or without knee support.

Needle type
Use 0.25 to 0.30 mm × 30 mm needle.

Needling directions
The muscle is identified using a pincer grip or flat palpation and needled in a superior to inferior direction.

Precautions
The deep lateral border of this muscle marks the path of the deep fibular nerve and the anterior tibial artery and vein.

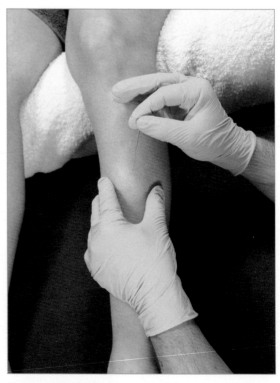

Supine with the knee supported.

FLEXOR DIGITORUM LONGUS

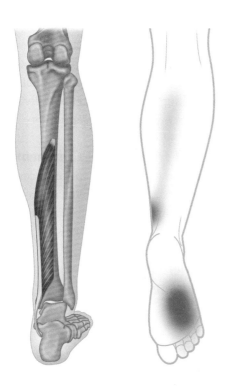

Latin, *flectere*, to bend; *digitorum*, of the toes; *longus*, long.

Origin
Medial part of the posterior surface of the tibia, below the soleal line.

Insertion
Bases of the distal phalanges of the second through fifth toes.

Nerve
Tibial nerve L5, S1, S2.

Action
Flexes all the joints of the lateral four toes (enabling the foot to firmly grip the ground when walking). Helps to plantar flex and invert the ankle joint.

Kinetic Chain Comment
Decelerates toe extension, foot dorsiflexion, and ankle eversion. An inhibited flexor digitorum longus can predispose the ankle or knee to soft tissue insult or lead to insult further up the kinetic chain.

Myofascial Trigger Point Comment
Flexor digitorum longus, accompanied by associated plantar muscles, causes pain and/or weakness in the foot and toes, with pain experienced particularly on the top or dorsal aspect of the foot and at times spreading to the anterior aspect of the tibia.

Practitioner Guidelines
Patient positioning
Patient is prone.

Needle type
Use 0.25 to 0.30 mm × 30 mm needle.

Needling directions
The muscle is identified and needled in a posterior to anterior direction.

Precautions
Avoid the tibial nerve and associated vessels.

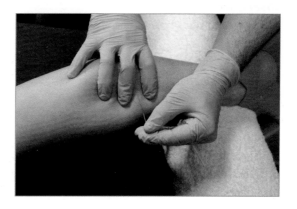

FLEXOR HALLUCIS LONGUS

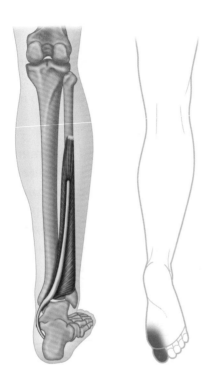

Latin, *flectere,* to bend; *hallucis,* of the great toe; *longus,* long.

Origin
Lower two-thirds of the posterior surface of the fibula, interosseous membrane, and adjacent intermuscular septum.

Insertion
Base of the distal phalanx of the great toe.

Nerve
Tibial nerve L5, S1, S2.

Action
Flexes all the joints of the great toe, playing a vital role in the final propulsive thrust of the foot during walking. Assists in plantar flexion and inversion of the ankle joint.

Kinetic Chain Comment
All foot and anatomical leg kinematic problems, structural or soft tissue related, can have adverse effects further up the kinetic chain, resulting in strain and eventually the formation of myofascial trigger points.

Myofascial Trigger Point Comment
Pain is referred to the great toe, mainly contained on the plantar surface, and is often mistaken for gout, as the pain is often described as a burning sensation, accompanied by stiffness.

Practitioner Guidelines
Patient positioning
Patient is prone.

Needle type
Use 0.25 to 0.30 mm × 30 mm needle.

Needling directions
Using flat palpation, locate and secure the myofascial trigger point within the palpable taut band. Insert the needle in a medial to lateral direction into the myofascial trigger point, toward or in the direction of the fibular bone.

Precautions
Avoid needling the neurovascular structures running in the posterior compartment.

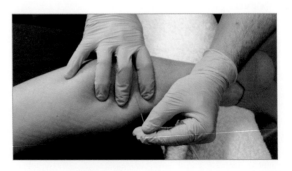

EXTENSOR HALLUCIS LONGUS

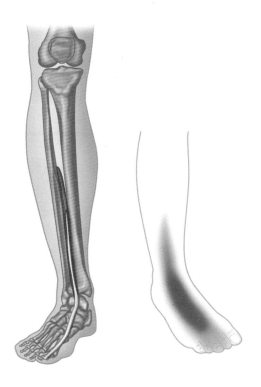

Latin, *extendere*, to extend; *hallucis*, of the great toe; *longus*, long.

Origin
Middle half of the anterior surface of the fibula, and adjacent interosseous membrane.

Insertion
Base of the distal phalanx of the great toe.

Nerve
Deep fibular nerve L4, L5, S1.

Action
Extends all the joints of the great toe. Dorsiflexes the ankle joint. Assists in inversion of the ankle joint.

Kinetic Chain Comment
Extensor hallucis longus is prone to spastic activity, which can lead to internal rotation of the fibula, resulting in kinematic changes up and down the kinetic chain.

Myofascial Trigger Point Comment
Pain and tenderness are experienced primarily on the plantar surface of the foot, with spillover pain on the plantar surface of the great toe. Often mistaken for gout or arthritis, this pain can be sharp and stinging, and can occasionally radiate up the kinetic chain for a short distance but does not extend to the heel.

Practitioner Guidelines
Patient positioning
Patient is prone, with the ankle supported.

Needle type
Use 0.25 to 0.30 mm × 30 mm needle.

Needling directions
For needling purposes, extensor hallucis longus lies between, and deep to, tibialis

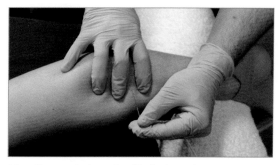

Needling technique for fibularis tertius or extensor hallucis longus.

anterior and extensor digitorum longus. The muscle is identified and needled in a superior medial to inferior lateral direction.

Precautions
The deep fibular nerve, along with its associated blood vessels, should be avoided by needling in a lateral to medial direction on the middle half of the anterior surface of the fibula. Tibialis anterior and the medial portion of extensor hallucis longus cover a portion of this neurovascular bundle, providing anatomical landmarks for safe needle application.

TIBIALIS POSTERIOR

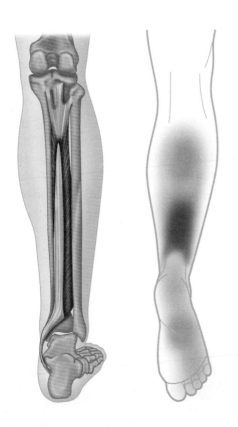

Latin, *tibialis*, relating to the shin; *posterior*, at the back.

Origin
Upper half of the lateral aspect of the posterior surface of the tibia, most of the interosseous membrane, and posterior fibula and fascia covering it posteriorly.

Insertion
Tuberosity of the navicular and plantar surface of the medial cuneiform. Tendinous expansions attach to the plantar surfaces of all the tarsal bones (except the talus), to the tip of the sustentaculum tali, and to the bases of the middle three metatarsals.

Nerve
Branch of the tibial nerve L4, L5, S1.

Action
Plantar flexes and inverts (supinates) the ankle. Eccentrically, decelerates subtalar joint pronation as it controls subtalar eversion and internal rotation of the tibia, and dynamically stabilizes the talonavicular joint. In the push-off phase of gait, assists in plantar flexion and inversion.

Kinetic Chain Comment
Tibialis posterior dives deep into the sole of the foot, the foundation upon which we all stand. Due to reciprocal inhibition, tibialis posterior can neurologically weaken, leading to compromised arch support. This can have implications further up the chain for links such as popliteus, posterior intermuscular septum, adductor magnus, and the core musculature.

Myofascial Trigger Point Comment

Most people will mistake the myofascial trigger points in tibialis posterior for Achilles tendinitis, plantar fasciitis, or shin splints. Pain is felt on the medial tibia or in the sole of the foot, at the level of the arch, when walking. Clients will often present with a pronated foot. A functional kinetic chain assessment is required, with appropriate activity to improve core stability and kinetic chain integrity.

Practitioner Guidelines

Patient positioning

Patient is prone, with the ankle supported.

Needle type

Use 0.25 to 0.30 mm × 30 mm needle.

Needling directions

The muscle is identified by dragging the medial gaster of gastrocnemius laterally using several fingertips and using the thumb as an axis. Palpate tibialis posterior deeper to soleus with the fingertips. Needle directly in and out across the frontal plane.

Precautions

Stay at the deep level of the tibial bone to ensure accuracy. The needle will also pierce a portion of the soleus muscle. This side approach will ensure that the needle does not enter the interosseous membrane.

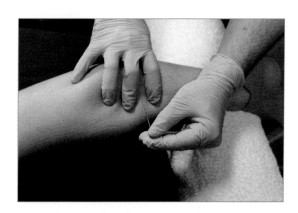

POPLITEUS

Latin, *poples*, the ham.

Origin

Anterior aspect of the lateral condyle of the femur, and oblique popliteal ligament of the knee joint. The muscle is anchored to the lateral condyle of the femur by a strong tendon, which passes into the capsule of the knee joint and can include the lateral meniscus.

Insertion

Posterior surface of the posterior side of the proximal tibia, above the soleal line.

Nerve

Tibial nerve L4, L5, S1.

Action

Medially rotates the tibia on the femur and flexes the knee (non-weight bearing). When the feet are fixed (closed-chain kinetics), laterally rotates the femur on the tibia and

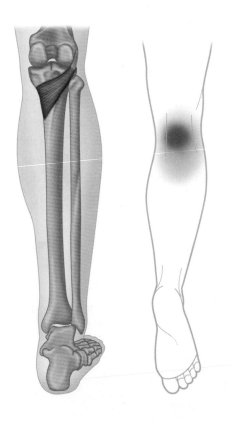

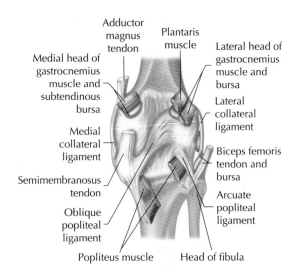

flexes the knee joint. Eccentrically, decelerates tibial rotation internally and femoral rotation externally (screw-home effect). Its function in posterolateral stability is significant.

Some anatomical papers describe a common idea of popliteus as a retractor of the lateral meniscus.

Kinetic Chain Comment
Machine-based exercise, such as prone leg curls, can overstress the popliteus, causing spasm and diminished screw-home capability. This, in turn, can lead to inhibition of the piriformis and deep hip rotators, with hyperextension at the knee. Shortness of popliteus can be confirmed by observing

slight flexion and internal rotation of the anatomical leg.

Myofascial Trigger Point Comment
Popliteus is a muscle that takes a lot of stressful abuse, and eventually myofascial trigger points can form, causing pain in the back of the knee. At night the pain reduces or ceases completely. Stiffness in the knee joint is often evident in the morning, with reduced ability to fully extend the anatomical leg.

On assessment, the foot can appear as if the leg has turned in (medial rotation at the knee). This is often a result of heavy squat exercises in the absence of appropriate neuromuscular stability at the joints and within the core.

Practitioner Guidelines
Patient positioning
Patient is prone, with the ankle supported. This muscle can also be targeted in a supine position, with the lower limb externally

rotated at the hip joint and the knee slightly flexed.

Needle type
Use 0.25 to 0.30 mm × 30 mm needle.

Needling directions
Direct the needle from the medial side, 20 mm below the knee, in an anterior and superior direction.

Precautions
This area is rich in neurovascular structures that are predominantly located in the midline. Working slowly will allow time for your patient to provide feedback concerning any nerve sensations due to the needle coming into the proximity of nerves, such as the saphenous or tibial.

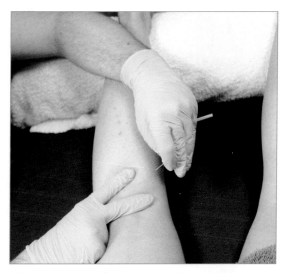

This muscle can also be targeted in a supine position, with the lower limb externally rotated at the hip joint and the knee slightly flexed.

FIBULARIS LONGUS

Latin, *fibula*, pin/buckle; *longus*, long. **Greek**, *perone*, pin/buckle.

Origin
Lateral condyle of the tibia (in conjunction with the extensor digitorum longus), upper two-thirds of the lateral surface of the fibula, intermuscular septa, and deep fascia.

Insertion
Plantar and lateral surface of the medial cuneiform, and base of the first metatarsal.

Nerve
Superficial fibular nerve L4, L5, S1.

Action
A foot evertor, fibularis longus assists in plantar flexing the ankle joint. Depresses the head of the first metatarsal. Eccentrically, decelerates ankle dorsiflexion and inversion of the subtalar joint during the push-off phase of gait.

Kinetic Chain Comment
Fibularis longus forms a sling or stirrup for the foot arches, offering an opposing force to tibialis anterior. Further up the kinetic chain, the muscle can affect the function of biceps femoris, sacrotuberous ligament, erector spinae, multifidus, etc.

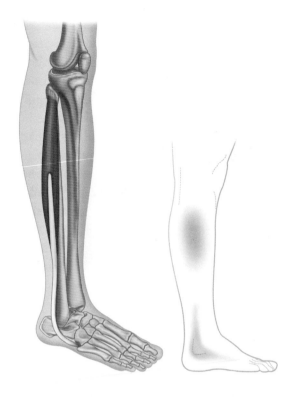

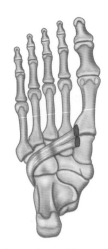

Insertion on base of first metatarsal
(plantar view, right foot)

Myofascial Trigger Point Comment

Along with fibularis brevis, myofascial trigger points refer pain down the leg over, above, and behind the lateral malleolus. Pain can also be felt over the anterolateral aspect of the ankle and the outside of the calcaneus. Many individuals with these myofascial trigger points complain of numbness or pins and needles in the toes, especially the third, fourth, and great toes.

Practitioner Guidelines

Patient positioning
Patient is prone, with the leg to be treated flexed and slightly externally rotated at the hip. The ankle of the treated leg is supported by a bolster.

Needle type
Use 0.25 to 0.30 mm × 30 mm needle.

Needling directions
Using flat palpation, locate and secure the myofascial trigger point within the palpable taut band. Insert the needle and direct it toward the lateral surface of the fibula.

Precautions
Avoid needling the common fibular nerve by needling 20 mm below the fibular head. Also avoid needling the superficial fibular and common fibular nerves.

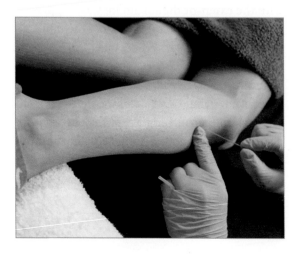

PLANTARIS

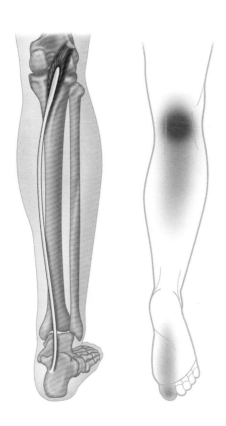

Latin, *plantaris*, relating to the sole.

Plantaris is a short, slender muscle and has the longest tendon in the body. Its origin is on the lateral supracondylar ridge, popliteal surface, and joint capsule. Inserting into the medial surface of the calcaneus, this muscle is a weak flexor of the knee and plantar flexes the ankle in the push-off phase of gait.

Plantaris is absent in about 10% of the population.

Origin
Inferior aspect of the lateral supracondylar line of the distal femur, and oblique ligament of the knee.

Insertion
Middle third of the posterior surface of the calcaneus, medial to the Achilles tendon.

Nerve
Tibial nerve L4, L5, S1.

Action
Plantar flexes the foot at the ankle, inverts the ankle, and assists in flexion at the knee.

Kinetic Chain Comment
Plantaris is a weak contributor to decelerating extension of the knee joint and decelerating eversion and dorsiflexion at the ankle.

Myofascial Trigger Point Comment
The pain from myofascial trigger points in plantaris mimics many pain syndromes firing into the posterior knee and down the medial aspect of the triceps surae into the heel, and sometimes into the ball of the foot and the great toe.

The therapist must rule out the possibility of S1 or S2 radiculopathy, rupture of the plantaris, popliteus tendinitis, tenosynovitis, popliteal artery aneurysm, Baker's cyst, deep vein thrombosis (DVT), intermittent claudication, peripheral vascular disease (PVD), avulsion of the popliteus tendon, muscle strain, posterior compartment syndrome, popliteal lymphedema, systemic infections or inflammation, nutritional inadequacy, metabolic imbalance, and toxicity and possible side effects of medications.

Practitioner Guidelines

Patient positioning
Patient is prone, with or without a bolster under the ankle, as appropriate.

Needle type
Use 0.25 to 0.30 mm × 30 mm needle.

Needling directions
The muscle is identified and needled in a superior medial to inferior lateral direction.

Precautions
Plantaris is only 2–4 in. (5–10 cm) long and is found on the medial border of the biceps femoris tendon. Palpate the inferior part of the lateral supracondylar ridge of the femur, just superior to the origin of the lateral head of the gastrocnemius. The popliteal artery, fibular nerve, and tibial nerve are to be avoided by directing the needle as shown in the image. Stay shallow and use a tangential approach.

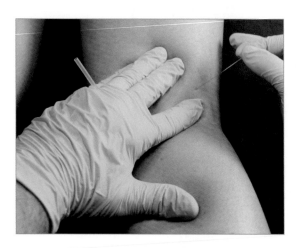

SOLEUS

Latin, *solea*, leather sole/sandal/sole (fish).

Lying deep to gastrocnemius, soleus is a broad, flat muscle resembling a flatfish.

Origin
Soleal line on the medial border of the tibia, posterior surface of the upper third of the fibula, and the fibrous arch between.

Insertion
By means of the calcaneal tendon to the middle part of the posterior surface of the calcaneus (heel bone).

Nerve
Tibial nerve L5, S1, S2.

Action
Plantar flexes the ankle, along with the gastrocnemius and plantaris.

Kinetic Chain Comment
From a dynamic postural viewpoint, soleus prevents the body falling forward at the ankle joint during standing. In gait, the muscle eccentrically decelerates subtalar joint pronation and internal rotation of the lower leg at heel-strike. It also decelerates dorsiflexion of the foot. Spasm or myofascial trigger points in soleus can be the origin of tight hamstrings, lower back pain, and even headaches.

Myofascial Trigger Point Comment
Soleus typically refers pain into the posterior aspect and plantar surface of the

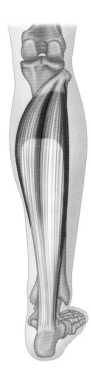

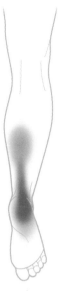

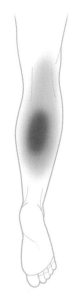

Referral pattern of TrPs in the area of the muscle slightly above a hand's width higher than the ankle crease

Referral pattern of TrPs in the gastrocnemius muscle bellies above the tendons

heel and to the distal end of the Achilles tendon. A rare myofascial trigger point spreads pain to the ipsilateral sacroiliac joint and can also refer pain to the jaw in extreme cases.

Practitioner Guidelines

Patient positioning
Patient is prone, with the ankle supported.

Needle type
Use 0.25 to 0.30 mm × 30 mm needle.

Needling directions
The muscle is accessed by targeting the area below gastrocnemius at the medial border of the tibia, and by moving the needle in a medial to lateral direction.

Precautions
Avoid the tibial nerve.

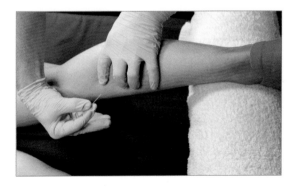

ABDUCTOR HALLUCIS

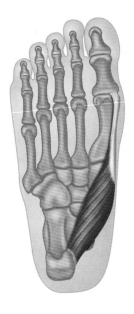
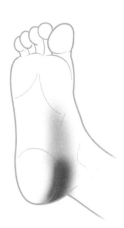

Latin, *abducere*, to lead away from; *hallucis*, of the great toe.

Origin
Along medial tuberosity of the calcaneal bone, flexor retinaculum, and plantar aponeurosis.

Insertion
By means of outer edge of the medial sesamoid, onto medial base of the proximal phalanx of the great toe (hallux).

Nerve
Medial plantar nerve L4, L5, S1.

Action
Abducts and flexes the metatarsophalangeal joint. Assists in adducting the forefoot.

Kinetic Chain Comment
Working with flexor hallucis brevis and longus and adductor hallucis longus (to control the great toe), abductor hallucis belongs to the first layer of muscles on the foot. It decelerates adduction of the hallux at the metatarsophalangeal joint (eccentric control toward the anatomical axis of the foot). Failure to do this leads to increasing pronation of the great toe and to the progression of the deformity.

Myofascial Trigger Point Comment
Pain is felt in the medial and posterior portions of the heel as well as in the instep. This pain can be experienced as a burning sensation on heel-strike and toe-off. Patients tend to limp into the clinic. Experience leads me to look at the footwear of a patient, which is often too small or fits poorly.

Be sure to rule out contributions from the possibility of L4 radiculopathy, S2 sciatic nerve lesion, Achilles tendinitis, plantar fasciitis, bone spur, pes cavus, pes planus (flat feet), bunions, congenital hypertrophy, Morton's foot syndrome, diabetic neuropathy, polyneuropathy, reflex sympathetic dystrophy, bone fracture, sprain/strain, tarsal tunnel syndrome, callus, involvements of blisters, bursitis, osteoarthritis, and rheumatoid arthritis. If in doubt, refer.

Practitioner Guidelines
Patient positioning
Patient is supine, with or without the knee supported by a bolster, as appropriate.

Needle type
Use 0.25 to 0.30 mm × 30 mm needle.

Needling directions
Needle in a superior to inferior direction and an anterior to posterior direction, moving the needle slowly and with care, and seeking feedback from the patient.

Precautions
Avoid placing the needle deep in the abductor hallucis, because numerous neurovascular structures (lateral plantar nerves) are located beneath the muscle.

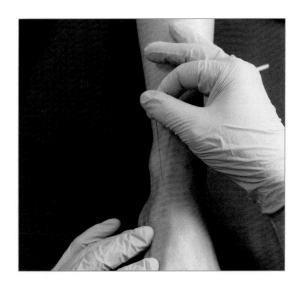

ADDUCTOR HALLUCIS

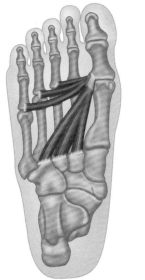
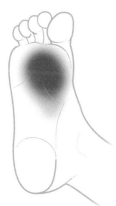

Latin, *adducere*, to lead to; *hallucis*, of the great toe.

Origin
Two heads (oblique and transverse) attach the adductor hallucis to the bases of the second to fourth metatarsal bones, plantar metatarsophalangeal ligaments of the third to fifth toes, and deep transverse metatarsal ligament.

Insertion
Lateral side of the base of the proximal phalanx.

Nerve
Lateral plantar nerve S1, S2.

Action
Adducts and assists in flexing the metatarsophalangeal joint of the great toe.

Kinetic Chain Comment
Implicated as a major deforming factor in hallux valgus, adductor hallucis decelerates movement of the proximal phalanx away from the second toe as well as the lateral sesamoid, thus reducing further pronation. Failure to do so adequately is a potent cause

of the more severe problem of hallux valgus deformity.

Myofascial Trigger Point Comment
The referral pattern is local, with pain felt on the distal sole under the metatarsal heads. Patients often report numbness. A frequently used patient description is a feeling of "fullness" in the area.

Practitioner Guidelines
Patient positioning
Patient is supine.

Needle type
Use 0.16 mm × 15 mm needle.

Needling directions
Needle in a superior to inferior direction, moving the needle slowly and with care, while seeking feedback from the patient.

Precautions
The foot is richly innervated, and the therapist must ensure that the correct needle gauge is used.

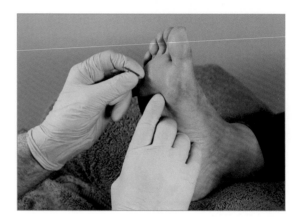

Glossary

Abductor	Muscle that moves a body part away from the midline of the body.
Acetylcholine (ACh)	Main neurotransmitter that is released in excessive amounts at affected motor endplates during the formation of myofascial trigger points as part of the Simons' Integrated Hypothesis.
Acetylcholinesterase	Biochemical that metabolizes acetylcholine.
Active scar	Any scar that is causing a symptom.
Active trigger point	Trigger point that causes pain when the muscle is in action or at rest.
Adductor	Muscle that moves a body part toward the midline of the body, thus adding to the midline.
Adenosine triphosphate (ATP)	Main cellular energy supplier.
Adhesion	Fibrous bands of normally separate tissues.
Adhesive capsulitis	Inflammatory thickening and adhesion of the tissues in the joint capsule, resulting in limitation of the range of motion.
Allodynia	Pain from a normally non-painful stimulus.
Anaerobic	Without oxygen.
Anterior	Pertaining to the front.
Aponeurosis	Flat form of tendon.
Antalgic gait	Unbalanced walking because of pain, with the weight spent most of the time on the less painful side during the stride.

Attachment trigger point	Trigger point occurring in a tendon or ligament or other attachment tissue, often initiated by the inflammatory reaction to sustained increased tension caused by trigger points in the more central parts of the muscle.
Axillary	Pertaining to the underarm or armpit.
Autonomic phenomena	Autonomic nervous system phenomena that may occur in the same general referral pattern as the pain pattern of a myofascial trigger point. Symptoms include blanching, redness, coldness, heat, redness, goosebumps, sweating, and hyper-secretion.
Barrier	Obstacle that prevents movement or access.
Belly (muscle)	Widest part of the muscle, also called a *gaster*.
Bilateral	Pertaining to two sides.
Biotensegrity	New way of understanding anatomy.
Bruxism	Clenching or grinding of the teeth.
Calcification	Process of tissue hardening by mineral salt deposition.
Cartilage	Firm, nonvascular type of connective tissue.
Cervicogenic	Generated in the neck.
Chronic	Longstanding or recurring, but not necessarily irreversible.
Composite pain pattern	Referral pattern from multiple, often overlapping, trigger points.
Contract–release	Gentle voluntary muscle contraction, immediately followed by a relaxation coupled with muscle lengthening through the normal physiological range of motion.
Contraction	Deliberate shortening of a muscle by electrical motor unit potentials (as opposed to a contracture).
Contraction nodule (or knot)	Nodules composed of clusters of trigger points.
Contracture	a sustained physiological muscle shortening in the absence of electrical motor unit potentials (as opposed to a *contraction*).
Core musculature	Muscles responsible for stabilizing the torso.
Dorsiflexor	Muscle that turns the foot or toes upward.

Dry needling	Use of a solid needle for pain therapy, rather than an injection of an anesthetic or other wet substance.
Dynamic	Pertaining to controlled movement, as opposed to a static state.
Dyspnea	Shortness of breath.
End plate	End of a motor nerve fiber.
Extensor	Muscle that increases the angle of a hinge joint.
Extraocular	Pertaining to outside the eye.
Extrinsic muscle	Muscle that originates outside the base structure and attaches to that structure.
Facet	Posterior vertebral joint, also called a *zygapophyseal joint*.
Facilitation	Process or activity that makes events more easily repeatable.
Failed surgical back	Symptoms remain or increase, in spite of back surgery.
Fascia	Three-dimensional integrative matrix that encloses and connects body structures, from the cellular level to the organ and muscle level.
Flexor	Muscle that reduces the angle of a hinge joint.
Foot drop and foot slap	Gait dysfunctions that describe the failure of the foot to clear the ground during the stride.
Gait	Manner of walking.
Gait cycle	Cycle of stride between the heel-strike of one foot and the next heel-strike of the same foot.
Gaster	Belly, as in the belly of a muscle.
Girdle (pelvic girdle, shoulder girdle)	Anatomically speaking, *girdle* refers to any structure that acts like a belt, e.g., the *shoulder girdle* refers to the bony ring and surrounding connective tissues that attach and support the shoulder.
Goniometer	Instrument that measures angles and is used in testing and documenting range of motion.
Hyperalgesia	Amplified pain reaction to a normally painful stimulus.
Hyperesthesia	Increased sensitivity to stimulation.

Hyperlax (or hypermobile)	Pertaining to a joint where movement occurs beyond the normal range expected.
Insulin resistance	Condition in which insulin is less and less able to metabolize glucose, and the body becomes resistant to the normal effect of insulin.
Intrinsic muscle	Muscle with both ends attaching to the base structure.
Involved muscle	Muscle with one or more myofascial trigger points.
Ischemic	Lack of oxygen rich, nutrient blood supply to meet current physiological needs of a cell, tissue, or organ.
Kinetic	Pertaining to movement or motion.
Kinetic chain	Anatomical chain of muscles and other tissue, linked through the fascia, that works together to produce movement.
Latent myofascial trigger point	Trigger point that causes pain when the muscle is in action.
Lateral	Pertaining to the side.
Local twitch response	Prolonged contraction of the taut band muscle fibers associated with a myofascial trigger point.
Lumbar	Pertaining to the lower back.
Matrix	Network.
Mediolateral	In the center to the side.
Monosynaptic reflex arc	"Reflex arc" is the path taken by the nerve impulses in a reflex action. In higher animals, most sensory neurons do not pass directly to the brain, but via a synapse in the spinal cord. "Monosynaptic" refers to the presence of a single chemical synapse.
Myalgia	Muscle pain.
Myofascia	Connective tissue (fascia) of the muscle.
Myofascial trigger point	Hyperirritable spot in skeletal muscle associated with a hypersensitive contraction nodule in a taut band.
Myogenic	Generated by muscle.

Neurotransmitter	Informational biochemical released from a cell to transfer a message across the gap to another cell.
Palpation	Act of touching with intent to diagnose or discover (taking a pulse is a form of palpation).
Paradoxical respiration	Form of breathing in which the chest expands and the belly contracts during the intake of breath. In healthy "belly breathing," the belly expands as the breath is drawn in, and contracts during exhalation.
Paresthesia	Abnormal sensations, including prickling, burning, tingling, or numbness.
Perineum	Area between the genitals and the anus.
Periosteum	Fibrous membrane covering the bone, except for the joint cartilage.
Plantar fasciitis	Inflammation of the plantar fascia.
Plantar flexor	Muscle that turns the foot or toes downward.
Posterior	Pertaining to the back.
Proprioception	Ability to recognize where one part of the body is in relation to other parts, and to the world around them.
Range of motion (ROM)	Distance that a joint can move from a flexed to an extended position. The *active* "ROM" is determined by the patient's muscle contraction. The *passive* "ROM" is generated by another person moving the muscles.
Receptor	Any type (sensory, motor, etc.) of nerve ending.
Referral pattern	Particular pattern of pain and/or other symptoms caused by a specific trigger point.
Rotoscoliosis	Scoliosis that includes a component of rotational curvature around the spinal column.
Sarcomere	Basic contractile unit of striated muscle.
Satellite trigger point	Trigger point formed due to the mechanical or neurogenic activity of another trigger point.
Sciatica	Lower back and hip pain that radiates down the back of the thigh into the calf. This is a description, not a diagnosis.

Scoliosis	Lateral spinal curvature.
Spasm	Increased muscle tension due to non-voluntary motor activity. It is not always accompanied by a shortening of the muscle.
Spillover pain	Increased area of referred pain and other symptoms that occurs in some patients because of greater hyper-irritability of a trigger point. It is more common, and often more extensive, in patients with multiple trigger points and central sensitization.
Static stretching	Stretching of a muscle while at rest, whereby the muscle is lengthened, and the stretch is held with no movement.
Taut band	Rope or string-like structure in a trigger-point-involved striated muscle.
Tinnitus	Ringing, crackling, or other unusual internally generated noises in the ear.
Trigeminal neuralgia	Condition that causes repeated (recurring) severe pains in parts of the face.
Trigger point cascade	Chain reaction that can occur when one trigger point activates and other muscles in the referral pattern, or those that compensate, activate satellites. At times this can be likened to a complex waterfall, with multiple trigger cascades occurring simultaneously.
Unilateral	Pertaining to one side.
Wide dynamic range (WDR)	Most abundant neuron with cell bodies located in the dorsal horn of the spinal cord.

Bibliography

Bishop, M.D., Beneciuk, J.M., and George, S.Z. 2011. Immediate reduction in temporal sensory summation after thoracic spinal manipulation. *Spine J* 11(5), 440–446 (doi. 10.1016/j.spinee. 2011.03.001).

Brisby, H. 2006. Pathology and possible mechanics of nervous system response to disc degeneration. *J Bone Joint Surg Am* 88(Suppl 2), 68–71.

Camanho, L.G., Imamura, M., and Arendt-Nielsen, L. 2011. Genesis of pain in arthrosis. *Revista Brasileira de Ortopedia* 46(1), 14–17.

Cotchett, M.P., Munteanu, S.E., and Landorf, K.B. 2014. Effectiveness of trigger point dry needling for plantar heel pain: A randomized controlled trial. *Phys Ther* 94(8), 1083–1094.

Cummings, M. 2003. Referred knee pain treated with electroacupunture to ilipsoas. *Acupunct Med* 21, 32–35.

Dommerholt, J. and Fernández-de-las-Peñas, C. 2013. *Trigger Point Dry Needling: An Evidence and Clinical-Based Approach*, London: Churchill Livingstone.

Dubousset, J. 2003. Spinal instrumentation: Source of progress but also revealing pitfalls. *Bull Acad Natl Med* 187(3), 523–533.

Edwards, J. 2005. The importance of postural habits in perpetuating myofascial trigger point pain. *Acupunct Med* 23(2), 77–82.

Fogelman, Y. and Kent, J. 2015. Efficacy of dry needling for treatment of myofascial pain syndrome. *J Back Musculoskel Rehab* 28(1), 173–179.

Fuller, R.B. 1961. Tensegrity. *Portfolio Art News Ann* 4, 112–127, 144, 148.

Gerwin, R.D., Dommerholt, J., and Shah, J. 2004. An expansion of Simons' integrated hypothesis of trigger point formation. *Curr Pain Headache Rep* 8(6), 468–475.

Gerwin, R., Shannon, S., Hong, C.Z., Hubbard, D., and Gervitz, R. 1997. Interrater reliability in myofascial trigger point examination. *Int Assoc Study Pain* 69(1–2), 65–73.

Giamberardino, M.A., Affaitati, G., Fabrizio, A., and Constantini, R. 2011a. Myofascial pain syndromes and their evaluation. *Best Pract Res Clin Rheumatol* 25(2), 185–198.

Giamberardino, M.A., Affaitati, G., Fabrizio, A., and Constantini, R. 2011b. Effects of treatment of myofascial trigger points on the pain of fibromyalgia. *Curr Pain Headache Rep* 15(5), 393–399.

Guimberteau, J.-C., Delage, J.-P., and Wong, J. 2010. The role and mechanical behavior of the connective tissue in tendon sliding. *Chirurgie de la Main* 29(3), 155–166.

Hsieh, Y.L., Chou, L.W., Joe, Y.S., and Hong, C.Z. 2011. Spinal cord mechanism involving the remote effects of dry needling on the irritability of myofascial trigger spots in rabbit skeletal muscle. *Arch Phys Med Rehab* 92, 1098–1105.

Hsueh, T.C., Yu, S., Kuan, T.S., and Hong, C.Z. 1998. Association of active myofascial trigger points and cervical disc lesions. *J Formos Med Assoc* 97(3), 174–180.

Huijing, P.A. 2009. Epimuscular myofascial force transmission: A historical review and implications for new research (International Society of Biomechanics Muybridge Award Lecture, Taipei, 2007). *J Biomech* 42(1), 9–21.

Kietrys, D.M., Palombaro, K.M., and Mannheimer, J.S. 2014. Dry needling for management of pain in the upper quarter and craniofacial region. *Curr Pain Headache Rep* 18(8), 437.

Koolstra, J.H. and van Eïjden, T.M. 2005. Combined finite-element and rigid-body analysis of human jaw joint dynamics. *J Biomech* 38(12), 2431–2439.

Kumaresan, S., Yoganandan, N., and Pintar, F.A. 1999. Finite element analysis of the cervical spine: A material property sensitivity study. *Clin Biomech* (Bristol, Avon) 14(1), 41–53.

Langevin, H. 2006. Connective tissue: A body-wide signaling network? *Med Hypotheses* 66(6), 1074–1077.

Levin, S. 1995. The importance of soft tissues for structural support of the body. *Spine: State of the Art Reviews* 9(2).

Lewit, K. 1979. The needle effect in the relief of myofascial pain. *Pain* 6(1), 83–90.

Lewit, K. and Kolar, P. 2000. Chain reactions related to the cervical spine. In: Murphy, D.R. (ed.), *Conservative Management of Cervical Spine syndromes*, New York: McGraw-Hill, 515–530.

Liu, Z.J., Yamagata, K., Kuroe, K., Suenaga, S., Noikura, T., and Ito, G. 2000. Morphological and positional assessment of TMJ components and lateral pterygoid muscle in relation to symptoms and occlusion of patients with temporomandibular disorders. *J Oral Rehabil* 27(10), 860–874.

Loeser, R.F. and Shakoor, N. 2003. Aging or osteoarthritis: Which is the problem? *Rheum Dis Clin North Am* 29(4), 653–673.

Lucas, K., Polus, B., and Rich, P. 2004. Latent myofascial trigger points: Their effects on muscle activation and movement efficiency. *J Bodywork Move Therap* 8, 160–168.

Lucas, N., Macaskill, P., Irwig, L., Moran, R., and Bogduk, N. 2009. Reliability of physical examination for diagnosis of myofascial trigger point: A systematic review of literature. *Clin J Pain* 25(1), 80–89.

Manheim, C.J. 1994. *The Myofascial Release Manual 2nd Edition*, Thorofare, NJ: Slack Inc., 124.

Martin, D.-C. and Levin, S. 2012. Myofascia as the tensioner in the biotensegrity model. In: Schleip, R., Findley, T.W., Chaitow, L. and Huijing, P.A. (2012).

Mayoral, O., Salvat, I., Martin, M.T., Martin, S., Santiago, J., Cotarelo, J., and Rodriguez, C. 2013. Efficacy of myofascial trigger point dry needling in the prevention of pain after total knee arthroplasty: A randomized, double-blinded, placebo-controlled trial. *Evid Based Complement Altern Med* 2013, 694941.

McMakin, C.R. 2011. *Frequency Specific Microcurrent in Pain*, Edinburgh: Churchill Livingstone Elsevier.

Mense, S. 2010. How do muscle lesions such as latent and active trigger points influence central nociceptive neurons? *J Musculoskelet Pain* 18, 348–353.

Modell, W., Travell, J.T., Kraus, H., et al. 1952. Relief of pain by ethyl chloride spray. *NY State J Med* 52, 1550–1558.

Moseley, G.L. 2012. Teaching people about pain: Why do we keep beating around the bush? *Pain Management* 2(1), 1–3.

Niddam, D.M., Chan, R.C., Lee, S.H., Yeh, T.C., and Hsieh, J.C. 2007. Central modulation of pain evoked from myofascial trigger points. *Clin J Pain* 23(5), 440–448.

Passerieux, E., Rossignol, R., Letellier, T., and Delage, J.P. 2007. Physical continuity of the perimysium from myofibers to tendons: Involvement in lateral force transmission in skeletal muscle. *J Struct Biol* 159(1), 19–28.

Reynolds, K.K., Ramey-Hartung, B., and Jortani, S.A. 2008. The value of CYP2D6 and OPRM1 pharmacological testing for opioid therapy. *Clin Lab Med* 28(4), 581–598.

Russell, I.J., Holman, A.J., Swick, T.J., et al. 2011. Sodium oxybate reduces pain, fatigue and sleep disturbance and improves functionality in fibromyalgia: Results from a 14-week, randomized, double-blind, placebo-controlled study. *Pain* 152(5), 1007–1017.

Samuel, A.N., Peter, A.A., and Ramanathan, K. 2007. The association of active myofascial trigger points with lumbar disc lesions. *J Musculoskel Pain* 15(2), 11–18.

Scarr, G. 2018. *Biotensegrity: The Structural Basis of Life, Second Edition*. Handspring Publishing: Edinburgh.

Schleip, R. and Müller, D.G. 2013. Training principles for fascial connective tissues: Scientific foundation and suggested practical applications. *J Bodywork Move Ther* 17(1), 103–115.

Schleip, R., Findley, T.W., Chaitow, L. and Huijing, P. A. (eds) 2012. *Fascia: The Tensional Network of the Human Body. The Science and Clinical Applications in Manual and Movement Therapies*, Edinburgh: Churchill Livingstone.

Shah, J.P. and Gilliams, E.A. 2008. Uncovering the biochemical milieu of myofascial trigger points using in-vivo microdialysis: An application of muscle pain concepts to myofascial pain syndrome, *J Bodywork Move Ther* 12(4), 371–384.

Shah, J.P. and Heimur, J. 2012. New frontiers in the pathophysiology of myofascial pain. *The Pain Practitioner* 2012, 26–32.

Sharkey, J. 2008. *The Concise Book of Neuromuscular Therapy*, Chichester: Lotus Publishing.

Sharkey, J. 2015. Biotensegrity-anatomy for the 21st Century. *Terra Rosa J* 16 <terrarosa.com.au>.

Sharkey, J. 2021. Fascia and tensegrity the quintessence of a unified systems conception. *Int J Anatomy and Applied Physiology*, 07(02), 174–178.

Simons, D.G. 2004. Review of enigmatic myofascial trigger points as a common cause of enigmatic musculoskeletal pain and dysfunction. *J Electromyogr Kinesiol* 14(1), 95–107.

Simons, D.G., Travell, J.G., and Simons, L.S. 1999. *Travell and Simons' Myofascial Pain and Dysfunction: The Myofascial Trigger Point Manual*, Vol. 1, 2nd edn, Baltimore, MD: Lippincott Williams & Wilkins.

Skorupska, E., Rychlik, M., Pawelec, W., Bednarek, A., and Samborski, W. 2014. Trigger point-related sympathetic nerve activity in chronic sciatic leg pain: A case study. *Acupunct Med* 32(5), 418–422.

Snapp, R.R., Goveia, E., Peet, L., Bouffard, N.A., Badger, G.J., and Langevin, H.M. 2013. Spatial organization of fibroblast nuclear chromocenters: Component tree analysis. *J Anat* 223(3), 255–261.

Soloman, L., Schnitzler, C.M., and Browett, J.P. 1982. Osteoarthritis of the hip: The patient behind the disease. *Ann Rheum Dis* 41(2), 118–125.

Srbely, J.Z., Dickey, J.P., Lee, D., and Lowerison, M. 2010. Dry needle stimulation of myofascial trigger points evokes segmental anti-nociceptive effects. *J Rehabil Med* 42(5), 63–68.

Staud, R. 2011. Peripheral pain mechanisms in chronic widespread pain. *Best Pract Res Clin Rheumatol* 25(2), 155–164.

Travell, J.G. and Simons, D.G. 1992. *Myofascial Pain and Dysfunction: The Myofascial Trigger Point Manual*, Vol. 2, Baltimore, MD: Lippincott Williams & Wilkins.

Willard, F. 2008. Basic mechanisms of pain. Future trends in CAM research in Integrative Pain Medicine: The Science and Practice of Complementary and Alternative Medicine. In: Audette, J.F. and Bailey, A. (eds), *Pain Management*, Totowa, NJ: Humana Press.

Woolf, C.W. 2010. Central sensitisation: Implications for the diagnosis and treatment of pain. *J Int Assoc Study Pain* 152(3), S2–S15.

Yates, B.J., Billig, I., and Cotter, L.A. 2002. Role of the vestibular system in regulating respiratory muscle activity during movement. *Clin Exp Pharmacol Physiol* 29(1–2), 112–117.

Yuan, M. et al. 2021. Pattern-recognition receptors are required for NLR-mediated plant immunity. *Nature*, 592(7852), 105–109.